SPECIAL PRAISE FOR
Out of the Woods

"Diane Cameron's stunning new book maps the territory of long-term recovery, acknowledging that the process at its best inexorably promotes the transformation of almost every area of life. *Out of the Woods* is an important achievement because it systematically explores territory that—remarkably enough—has simply not been mapped in any serious fashion. We're fortunate that it was Cameron who undertook this important task—fortunate in no small part because she is a superb writer. Her voice radiates the maturity of long-term recovery, never doctrinaire, lively, fun, inspiring, engaging, and nonreactive, but relentlessly challenging stale assumptions wherever she finds them. I predict this book will soon be on the night-tables (and in the purses) of untold numbers of recovery explorers!"

—STEPHEN COPE
DIRECTOR, KRIPALU INSTITUTE FOR EXTRAORDINARY LIVING
AUTHOR OF *The Great Work of Your Life*

"Diane Cameron has illuminated the special challenges and opportunities that women with several decades of addiction recovery share, and has brought the wisdom of that journey to all who decide to get on that path.

"She shows what it takes to stay in recovery as you weather financial, sexual, professional, and interpersonal challenges, and she shows that while you don't need to worry about relapse all the time, there are always new things you can explore to become the best version of yourself."

—CAROLINE ADAMS MILLER
MASTER OF APPLIED POSITIVE PSYCHOLOGY (MAPP)
AUTHOR OF *My Name Is Caroline* AND *Creating Your Best Life*

"With the clear-eyed view of a woman with over thirty years in recovery, Diane Cameron's *Out of the Woods* is like an intimate conversation with a wise and loving sponsor. She shares the tools of the Twelve Steps in ways that speak to women in long-term recovery, who are dealing with life changes, body changes, an evolving spirituality, and an expanding sense of service to a larger community."

—AMY WEINTRAUB
FOUNDER OF LIFEFORCE YOGA
AUTHOR OF *Yoga for Depression* AND *Yoga Skills for Therapists*

OUT
of the
WOODS

OUT of the WOODS

A WOMAN'S GUIDE to LONG-TERM RECOVERY

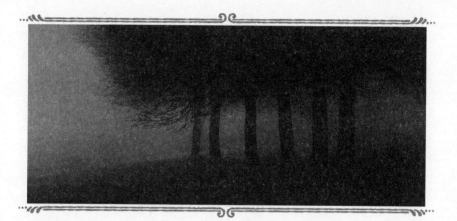

Diane Cameron

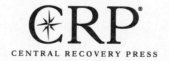

CENTRAL RECOVERY PRESS

Las Vegas

Central Recovery Press (CRP) is committed to publishing exceptional materials addressing addiction treatment, recovery, and behavioral healthcare topics, including original and quality books, audio/visual communications, and web-based new media. Through a diverse selection of titles, we seek to contribute a broad range of unique resources for professionals, recovering individuals and their families, and the general public.

For more information, visit www.centralrecoverypress.com.

Publisher: Central Recovery Press
      3321 N. Buffalo Drive
      Las Vegas, NV 89129

19 18 17 16 15 14   1 2 3 4 5

ISBN: 978-1-937612-47-4 (paper)
       978-1-937612-48-1 (e-book)

Sharon Zukin, *Point of Purchase: How Shopping Changed American Culture*. New York: Routledge, 2004, p.112. Used with permission.

Publisher's Note: This book contains general information about recovery and related matters. The information is not medical advice, and should not be treated as such. Central Recovery Press makes no representations or warranties in relation to the information in this book. If you have any specific questions about any medical matter discussed in this book, you should consult your doctor or other professional healthcare provider. This book is not an alternative to medical advice from your doctor or other professional healthcare provider.

Our books represent the experiences and opinions of their authors only. Every effort has been made to ensure that events, institutions, and statistics presented in our books as facts are accurate and up-to-date. To protect their privacy, the names of some of the people, places, and institutions in this book have been changed.

Cover design and interior design and layout by Marisa Jackson

THIS BOOK IS DEDICATED TO THE
ANONYMOUS PROGRAMS IN GRATITUDE
FOR THE MIRACLE OF RECOVERY.

*"Give freely of what you find and join us.
We shall be with you in the Fellowship of the Spirit . . . ."*

TABLE of CONTENTS

Introduction

IN MANY TWELVE-STEP PROGRAMS newcomers are either consoled or chastened by being told that it can take three to five years to "get out of the woods." It's a way of saying that recovery takes time. Later, at about the five-year mark, after attending a considerable number of meetings and working the steps and making countless life changes, many of us realize that it has actually taken that long simply to get *into* the woods. It is there—to continue the woodsy metaphor— that we start to recognize the trees and to know the creatures and critters of the woods for what they are.

Then the near-magical thing happens. Long-term recovery begins to take hold. Slowly, especially for women, there is a sensation of coming out of the woods. It's a sense that we absolutely have changed, that there is some stability in our lives, and that we are truly new people. Of course we are not "fixed" and we're never "cured," but in double-digit recovery, another kind of life begins. And it remains, even after ten or fifteen or more years, to be about "progress, not perfection."

After ten years of meetings and working the Twelve Steps, recovery often shifts into a different pace and schedule. This can be baffling to people in other stages of recovery and it can be troubling to those who are at that ten-plus place: What does it mean that I go to fewer meetings? Why am I spending more time on other projects, people, and other kinds of personal development? What does it mean to be a recovering woman in double-digit recovery?

There are larger numbers of us in recovery. And a surprising number of us have been around for more than ten years, but we don't always speak up about what happens. I have come to believe that we need to share our perspective.

The number of women who began to attend various twelve-step programs in the 1980s created a significant demographic bump. Those women are reaching key milestones now. Today, women are coming into twelve-step programs in ever growing numbers. The National Council on Alcoholism and Drug Dependencies (NCADD) estimates that women make up more than 35 percent of the Alcoholics Anonymous (AA) membership and more than 45 percent of Narcotics Anonymous (NA) membership. In Overeaters Anonymous (OA) and Al-Anon and Adult Children of Alcoholics (ACOA) that number is closer to 75 percent. There are larger numbers of us in recovery. And a surprising number of us have been around for more than ten years, but we don't always speak up about what happens. I have come to believe that we need to share our perspective.

At the five-year mark we start to get a sense of what is truly ours and what belongs to other people, or to the past. We begin to have new habits, new skills, and new friends. Working the steps and learning from others takes us through layers of self-examination. We begin to grow up.

Our spiritual growth starts to dovetail with our psychological work. We begin to look at our careers, our relationships, and our spirituality. We find spiritual practices that work for us. In years seven to nine we "dig deep or die" and recommit to our recovery. At ten years we have rich lives, and we work to balance our life in "the rooms" with the rest of our life.

We are coming out of the woods.

So why make a point of the ten-year mark in recovery? Why a special book for women who've been recovering for ten or more years? Because while the basics remain the same, some issues are different after you have been in recovery for a while. Most women with long-term recovery have a sense of this. There are situations we mention or describe in the rooms and the details we share only with recovering friends. And we *have* good friends. One of the striking phenomena about later recovery is that we even have friends who are not in recovery—*and who don't need to be.*

Yes, we still struggle, and no, we're not perfect by a long shot. If we're lucky and we have a sense of humor—that grows over time, too—we've given up any hope of perfection and we've come to have a comfortable relationship with our flaws and with ourselves.

What most of us have learned is that the Twelve Steps and a recovery program are part of a good life, but that even recovery does not protect us from illness, job troubles, problems with our kids or family, and experiencing all types of losses. We, like everyone else, will get to experience plenty of "life on life's terms."

RECOVERY IS A SUBTLE GAME

My favorite bumper sticker has always been, "I didn't quit, I surrendered," and I love sayings like, "Give time time," and "Trust the process." But now, with nearly thirty years in twelve-step recovery, I feel a kind of nostalgia that time has indeed passed and that the doors that opened so generously years ago to welcome me into a twelve-step fellowship now open again and deliver me—drug-free, sane, *and* still healing—back into the world. It's like riding in one of those elevators with doors that open on either end. You get in, and it goes up or down, but you have to turn around and face the other way to get out. That is what it feels like to be a woman in recovery coming out of the woods.

Long-term recovery has a kind of ease and grace to it.
That is what the newcomers are seeing
when they "want what you have."

Of course this doesn't mean we graduate. Nor do we leave recovery. But it's different. Long-term recovery has a kind of ease and grace to it. That is what the newcomers are seeing when they "want what you have." Not that there aren't days that I hurt like hell, or act like a brat, or suffer with emotional pain. The difference is that on those days—like the day my brother died or when I learned that my husband was seriously ill—even then, as I was lying on the floor and crying, there was a part of me that could watch myself do that and say, "Go ahead, cry; you will be okay."

That's another plus of long-term recovery: I no longer automatically assume when something bad happens that I did something wrong or that I am being punished.

Years ago, before I came into the rooms of recovery, when something bad happened it was likely that it did have to do with something I'd done. I drank to excess, lied about it, made crummy decisions, and drank more to tolerate the shame and guilt. I swung back and forth between compulsive work and sloth, tried bulimia and compulsive eating, got into financial trouble, and made a mess of most relationships.

I remember going to see a therapist in those painful days before my recovery began. She listened to me pour out my pain, asked a few questions, and then looked me in the eye and told me that I would need to be in therapy for about three years. I left her office in tears. She did get through my defenses but I felt hopeless about her prescription. How could I possibly do anything for three years?

Then one day at work I heard some women gossiping about a woman I admired. I didn't know her well, but she seemed smart and kind and had a refreshing sense of humor. The women at work were whispering, "Well, you know she goes to AA." I know they thought they were saying something awful about her, but I thought, "Oh my God, she goes to AA . . . and she's so pulled together . . . she goes to AA!" It was my first experience of "If you want what we have . . . ," and I hadn't even been to a meeting yet.

I think of that day whenever I hear someone say, "You may be the only Big Book someone reads." That gossip was a gift. It was the first of many experiences in recovery where something bad, like listening to gossip, turned out to have a higher purpose.

So I went to my first recovery meeting. In a church basement of course, and the rest is history—or my history, actually. I remember how in those first months I would hear people with three or five years talking about their lives and "working a program." I could see that they had decent lives; they smiled and laughed and seemed to be moving forward.

Some of them had been in recovery for many years. It seemed impossible, but in that way that recovery happens—one-day-at-a-time, and spending so many hours sitting on folding chairs and drinking coffee—one day I had ten years. My gratitude was inexpressible. My life was new in almost every way; my faith in the recovery process absolute.

But in these later years, I have begun to have new questions and different ideas. There are life issues that no one talked about when I was younger in recovery. It seems that when I look around I see fewer of "us"; people with ten or more years are harder to find. Does it mean that we relapse or we simply drift away after ten years? Does it suggest a lack of commitment or gratitude?

When I look closer though, that is not what I see happening.

I am gifted with a group of women friends who have between ten and thirty years of recovery. Sometimes when we have dinner or we take walks together we talk about these changes in our recovery. We share about the tools we still use and those that we depend on less now. We talk about what has stayed the same and what hasn't. When I take a close look at these friends, and myself, I see happy, busy women. Like another recovery slogan says, "Recovery didn't just save my life; it gave me a life worth saving." And that is now truer than ever.

The good news is that with double-digit recovery there often is less pain. The bad news is that pain was what motivated us toward change and continued spiritual growth.

I notice how subtle recovery can be. After a period of ten years we are different people. The big glaring chunks of our disease have been removed. We look better both inside and out. Sometimes we tell stories about what we struggle with today—yes; struggle remains as long as we are committed to growth. "Progress not perfection" is the slogan of choice. There are rewards that begin to come true with ten or more years of recovery, but those specific rewards sometimes take us away from the people and practices that built our good recovery.

The good news is that with double-digit recovery there often is less pain. The bad news is that pain was what motivated us toward change and continued spiritual growth. So what is a recovering woman to do? And what does remain? I think the answer is in more questions and more vigilance.

In earlier stages of recovery our shifts of mind and changes of attitude were mirrored by external changes. We saw people gain or lose weight, or cut and color their hair. We dressed differently, dated differently, took jobs, quit jobs, changed career fields, got married and got divorced, and sometimes got married again. The changes were obvious and dramatic. If you laid the photos of our first year next to the photos from years five and seven and ten, you could see women change. It shows on the outside, but if we could X-ray the minds and hearts of women in later recovery we'd see that dramatic change continues, but now more than ever, it's an inside job.

In later recovery we find our stride and our style. The work we do is less obvious from the outside. Now it's not so much about losing weight or getting a promotion or a diploma. We've learned to incorporate self-care; we can be decent coworkers; we've changed careers or gone back to school. Now maybe it's about being kinder and not about being the smarty-pants; it's about taking pride in our work and not needing applause—or even better, now we can be the one who applauds others. It's more about what we *don't* do than what we do.

ALL THESE YEARS AND YOU ARE STILL NOT ALONE

What women in recovery for ten or more years have is a set of skills and a wealth of experience to fall back on. We recognize our patterns, we can cut through our defenses sooner, and we learn not to fight the inevitable. We learn to surrender when we see the wall coming at us instead of waiting, as we did in the past, to slam right into it.

We are also able to see those difficult circumstances that we find ourselves in with a tiny bit more perspective. By the time we reach the ten-year mark, most of us have had at least one or two experiences of having something we were sure wasn't supposed to happen turn out to be the stepping stone to something unexpectedly good.

Life at ten-plus years can have its challenges. This book was written by a woman for women with ten or more years of recovery. To help us compare notes, to see that there is common ground, and to reassure us that there is no one right way to be a recovering woman. I hope to enhance your recovering lives and offer you markers along the path as you grow out of the woods.

Chapter One

STAGES of RECOVERY

WHEN WE WERE "YOUNGER" IN recovery we heard the warnings about focusing on the length of time someone has in recovery. Statements like "The person who got up earliest this morning is the one with the most recovery," or "All anyone has is these twenty-four hours." We were cautioned that we should not be lulled into false security by the number of years we had in recovery, nor overly impressed by the number of candles on anyone else's anniversary cake. We were told, "While you are in meetings, your disease is in the corner doing push-ups," or "The longer you are in recovery the closer you are to using." These sayings were intended to remind us that we should not put too much stock in numbers. We were warned against hubris and pride. But while it is true that "all anyone has is these twenty-four hours," it is also true that our learning accrues, and there is a reason we listen carefully to the old timers. For although there is danger, there is also wisdom in the woods. Those with long-term recovery have eluded many of those dangers and have collected much of the wisdom.

When we were new to recovery we measured time much like parents do with a new baby. We gave our recovery "age" in numbers of days or weeks or months until we turned two and then we started counting years. In those "younger" years of recovery, someone who had been around longer probably said to us, "It will take you three to five years to get out of the woods," and we wondered how we'd ever survive.

But we begin to grow up. We make friends, develop new habits, and practice new skills. Working the steps and listening to others takes us through layers of self-examination. As we closed in on that crucial five-year mark we realized that while we did have more stability and a new set of habits, that "edge of the woods" we'd been expecting was still a long way off.

At the five-year point we understand that it takes five years simply to get into the woods. We see our own patterns and know our true feelings. We can discern what belongs to our own personality.

If we have a good sponsor and a close circle of recovering friends, the five-year mark is a perfect time to take another Fourth Step inventory, assuming we have done one already. We get to do a deeper one here because we may have avoided doing one that includes the positives or assets. Typically, in our first inventory we are relieved to give away secrets and things we feel shame about. But later we realize that a true inventory must include what is good and valuable as well.

At five years, as we look around these woods, we can see that we do have talents and strengths. It gets easier, though never easy, to claim those strengths along with our defects.

At five years our spiritual growth starts to dovetail with our psychological work. We look at our careers and relationships. We find a spiritual practice that works for us.

In years seven to nine we "dig deep or die," as the old timers say. This is a time when we have to recommit to recovery. If we stay in the process we keep growing. Yes, we still have problems and struggles, but we learn more about ourselves with each year. Around year seven we often become leaders in our groups. We have knowledge and experience to give back and we do it willingly. We chair meetings and coordinate conferences. We attend and sometimes lead retreats; we are trusted servants in our home group and maybe also in our regions.

Typically in this stage, our lives outside of our recovery program are growing as well. Our careers develop; our kids grow up or maybe we have a new family. We become better parents.

We reclaim relationships with our own family. We find ourselves welcome at holidays and sometimes we are the hosts for special family events. Humor returns for us and for those around us. We can be trusted now. Enough of our amends are done so that we can laugh when we talk about the past with those who witnessed it up close. Our lives are rich and full.

At ten or fifteen years we have truly rich lives both in and out of "the rooms," and now we have to balance "the rooms" with the rest of our lives.

We also now understand, in a new way, that there is no secret contract with God and no special deal for people in recovery. Yes, we are special because we have the gift of recovery but we are, at the same time, not so special.

We finally get it that we absolutely don't have control. The things that happen to other women will happen to us:

trouble with children, problems at work, financial difficulties, divorce, betrayal, cancer, disabilities, and people we love will die and we will grieve hard.

Recovery cannot spare us those things. Recovery doesn't keep us from being touched by human life. We understand—quietly and seriously—that this is real life. And we'll take it, and we say thank you.

THE COLORS OF RECOVERY WILL CHANGE

When I celebrated my fifth year of recovery, my friend Miriam made a quilted wall hanging for me to mark that significant anniversary. Miriam was ahead of me in recovery and she had celebrated her twelfth anniversary. Quilting was one of the passions that she'd reclaimed thanks to recovery and she was, much to her own surprise, very good at it.

The quilt panel that she made for me she called "Stages of Recovery." It is a vertical panel that links four quilted squares on a deep burgundy background. The panels represent four stages of recovery and they begin at the top with a distinct checkerboard of black-and-white panels. This top square, Miriam told me, represents the start of recovery and the black-and-white necessity of not using your addictive substance or behavior. The stark contrast is about following the rules and doing what you are told. The black-and-white color scheme is clearly, "On/Off" and "Good/Bad."

The panel below that one is another square with a strong black base and side columns of pure white, but with a deep pink band across the top that dips down to touch the back squares.

"This is your pink cloud phase," Miriam said. "This is where you are so happy to be in recovery; things are starting to get better; you see the gifts of the program and you just want more."

I do remember that time of my recovery well. I talked about recovery to everyone. I carried recovery books and pamphlets home with me for the holidays. What? Not a table topic for Thanksgiving? This is the time when some of us begin to proselytize. We are so proud of ourselves that we break our own anonymity, and we can't understand why everyone isn't following our lead and joining a twelve-step program. Life is going to be fantastic from now on, right? Alas.

The next square down on my "stages" quilt is a square that includes neat rectangles made of black and white and pink prints. It's pretty but not regimented like the stark black-and-white square at the top. This third square has something new: Now there are also deep gray squares scattered among the printed ones and a solid charcoal gray square at the exact center.

Yes, this represents that the gray of recovery and the gray of life have arrived.

The last quilt square is the shocker. The bottom piece is made up of many small squares seemingly tossed at random. Some are the now-familiar black and white and pink ones and there's even some gray, but mixed in are more squares of candy red, bright blue, acid green, deep purple, tangerine orange, and a dull mustard yellow. There is no order in this stage. This square is distractingly messy, but it is deeply and happily colorful.

For years I disliked that last square. The other sections with their deliberate and limited palettes were graphic and sharp—and orderly—but this last square with its messy mix of too many colors always bothered me. But that bottom square signifying the "messy but colorful" part of recovery is what *Out of the Woods* is all about: messy progress, happiness, not perfection.

What we know now is that, as women in recovery, we need each of these stages and we need them in this order. When we are new, we need to submit to and embrace strict rule-following. "Don't use—no matter what." "If your ass falls off, pick it up and take it to a meeting."

Then, as recovery starts to take, we are embraced in and humored through our "pink clouds," but they too run their courses. The gray enters our recovery and we find that it's a time when working with a sponsor and good recovery friends matter.

Discernment is a skill we have to develop in these gray years. Our recovery becomes our own; we make choices based on recovery principles, but our choices may not look like anyone else's.

Then, if we keep coming around and we keep growing, our lives become more colorful and yes, even messy. This is when we have to figure out what our recovery will be like for the long haul. This may also be the time when newcomers or people in the black-and-white stages will question or challenge our commitment. They might say things like, "If you don't go to three meetings a week you are going to use."

Those in their own pink cloud stages will wonder at our suffering or our struggles. "She must not be working a good program if she is sad." Or "She needs to practice the Third Step and everything will turn out fine." They will want to believe that if they get their recovery "just right"—kind of like Goldilocks—then they will be spared the realities of human life that everyone experiences as we age.

Finally, in that colorful and messy stage, we will have fewer "shoulds." We might have a sponsor or a few close recovering women friends. We might leave the marriage that in early recovery we worked so hard to save. We might have a baby—with or without a partner. We might leave our law practice to be an artist while our best friend gives up her successful pottery business to go to nursing school. There are no right answers. Plenty of confusion and new problems appear for sure, but we are guided through these times by a strong foundation of deep recovery.

As a newcomer I was attracted to those who looked good on the outside—often those who spoke well, were successful at work, and seemed to have it all together.

WHO HAS WHAT YOU WANT?

In early recovery I heard this advice over and over: "Look for someone who has what you want, and ask them how they got it." That was also the advice I was given for how to pick a sponsor. As a newcomer I was attracted to those who looked good on the outside—often those who spoke well, were successful at work, and seemed to have it all together. But when I look around the rooms today, it's not always the shiny stars or fine talkers who have what I want.

I started thinking about this when I was trying to encourage a woman I sponsored to do more step work. "But I'm not using my drugs of choice, and I don't feel like I want to use them," she told me. I tried to tell her that I want so much more than only abstinence from my recovery.

It's true; I want more than abstinence from alcohol or other drugs or behaviors. I want more than a saner schedule or a good marriage. I want the whole enchilada. I want a deeply changed mind and heart, and I want peace, serenity, and joy. I also want the highest quality relationships possible—with my husband, family, friends, my higher power of course, and, yes, with myself.

But here's where it gets tricky. That good, changed life comes with longevity; more time in recovery does equal more exposure to new ideas, concepts, and learning as we go, layer upon layer, through the Twelve Steps. But those changes and that growth are not directly correlated to simply accumulating days in recovery. And not everyone in the rooms wants the kind of deep, continual life-changing recovery that I am describing. I find that I still have to look around the rooms and ask myself, "Who has what I want?"

It's possible to have thirty-five years of recovery and still be miserable and unhappy and filled with resentment and fear. (Sorry, but it's true.) We share the rooms with some people who have been around a long time and they are still unhappy at work and unhappy in their primary relationships. That is not the kind of recovery I seek. I want a quality recovery. Marty Mann, one of the first women to recover in Alcoholics Anonymous, and a close friend of Bill Wilson, is credited with first expressing the notion that it's the quality of your recovery that counts, not the length of it.

TWIGS* FOR CHAPTER ONE:
Stages of Recovery

- What is your image for the stages of your recovery?
  A quilt? Map? Ladder? Tree? Can you draw, paint,
  or collage it?

- Divide your recovery into five-year blocks. Name each
  one as if it were a movie or a song.

- Write in your journal about something you "knew for
  sure" in your first few years. Is that still true? What
  changed and what hasn't?

*One of the definitions of *twig* is to comprehend the meaning of; so in keeping with the woods analogy, I thought I would offer these *twigs* to help you further understand what I shared in the chapter.

Chapter Two

PHYSICAL: BRING the BODY

ONE DAY, MANY YEARS AGO, I woke up with a terrible pain in my back. I didn't remember doing anything in particular to cause it but the pain was bad. I went to a chiropractor and I expected him to fix my back. I thought he'd make a few adjustments and I'd be all better.

The doctor did an examination, and then he had me walk and move and sit and stand up and sit down again while he watched. He had me try some stretches to test my flexibility. And he made notes. He did a few adjustments and then we sat and talked. He talked to me about how I sat and stood and moved. We talked about my writing and reading and my sleeping habits, and how I drove my car.

He explained that I had not hurt my back overnight. The injury had been a slow process of incremental habits building up to cause weakness in some areas of my body and overcompensation of certain other muscles, and to my impatient dismay, my healing would follow the same course: I would have to incorporate new habits over a long period of time.

The doctor told me I would need to change my desk and my chair and also my steering wheel and my pillow—all of which would feel uncomfortable at first because I was used to the unhealthy habits. I would have to learn new ways of sitting, standing, and driving, and by doing that—and doing it over time—my weak muscles would get stronger and my misused muscles would realign.

We start with the physical. Our addiction has almost always caused physical damage—whether it is from drinking, smoking, eating, sex, or other behavioral/process aspects of our disease like television or technology; there is almost always injury to our physical health.

He explained that my back would recover as I learned these new movement patterns, and that I would have to practice them until they became second nature. The repair and healing would come from small, incremental changes over time.

It was much like my recovery from my addiction.

Addiction is a three-part illness (body, mind, and spirit), and it requires a three-part recovery. We start with the physical. Our addiction has almost always caused physical damage—whether it is from drinking, smoking, eating, sex, or other behavioral/process aspects of our disease like television or technology—there is almost always injury to our physical health.

So our recovery began with the physical too. We stopped using, drinking, hurting ourselves with food or work or cigarettes or worry. Then as our recovery progressed, we learned to continue with our physical care. We stopped smoking, lost weight, started to exercise, took yoga classes, or learned to dance. We went to healthcare practitioners (and we followed their advice) and we stopped procrastinating about the dentist, the gym, and learned to eat better.

If we were to take a look in the medicine cabinets of women with more than ten years of recovery, we can see there's no "one-right-way." Yes, again, the colorful, messy stage.

One recovering woman may have a bare medicine cabinet with only Band-Aids and aspirin. Another recovering woman looks like she's got the local pharmacy in her cabinet, although a closer look reveals nonnarcotic and nonalcoholic cough medicine, anti-inflammatories, antidepressants, and tubes of different antibiotic salves. For this woman, these medicines are health remedies and they are used strictly according to directions. In yet another recovering woman's medicine cabinet you'll find Chinese herbs, vitamins A to Z, St. John's Wort, arnica cream, and Bach Flower remedies; for her it's all about natural choices. And still others may feel that even an herbal remedy is off limits for their recovery.

LOOKING GOOD AND FEELING GOOD

At some point in recovery most women begin to take better care of their bodies. It's a natural progression. Maybe dieting didn't work before because we were drinking half of our daily calorie allotment, as well as eating. Or maybe we had to stop jogging in early recovery because our exercise compulsion was out of control. But at some point in our double-digit years we'll begin to look at diet, exercise, and our overall health.

We also find that as our life gets better we want to have more energy to enjoy that life and enjoy it longer. That too will lead us to pay attention to nutrition, fitness, and preventative healthcare. We know that becoming physically strong can increase our psychological strength as well. Most of us have seen the articles and news reports that detail the research showing that regular exercise can help us to manage stress. Women in recovery—who may have a variety of additional stressors—can benefit especially.

MEDICATION USE

An important part of taking care of our bodies is being mindful of medications. This is always a tricky area for people in recovery, and as people in long-time recovery we have to be *especially* aware. It's possible that the longer we are in recovery, the more comfortable we become, and the more "normal" we may feel, especially with issues around healthcare and medicines.

It's also true that the longer we are in recovery, the older we are, and that simple fact of aging means additional health-related issues. Now, I'm not a doctor and even the doctors we meet as comrades in recovery are not experts on medications for recovering people. We need to turn to true experts—our own physicians who know about our history of addiction, or doctors who specialize in addiction medicine.

For example, most of us avoid the class of medicines called benzodiazepines (or benzos, in slang parlance). Benzos include Valium, Xanax, Ativan, Klonopin, Librium, etc., and are often prescribed for anxiety or depression. Any usage should be only at need, and then strictly supervised by a doctor who knows us and knows of our addiction.

Also to be avoided are prescription painkillers and other opioid-based drugs: morphine, methadone, Vicodin, Oxycontin, Percocet, Dilaudid, Lortab, etc. A trip to the dentist can lead to disaster for a person in recovery who takes these, even as directed, unless strict precautions are taken.

Aging bodies can lead to new hips, new knees, and back surgeries. And those often come with the need for temporary use of serious pain medications.

We must beware of stimulants, as well. Illegal ones include cocaine and meth, of course, but also prescriptions, such as Ritalin and Concerta. Even some over-the-counter asthma medications have a stimulating effect. There is even some controversy in twelve-step circles over the use of so-called "energy drinks," or excessive caffeine consumption.

We also want to be careful even as we face the good news of better medicine. Aging bodies can lead to new hips, new knees, and back surgeries. And those often come with the need for temporary use of serious pain medications. We have all known people in long-term recovery who have been led to relapse by correctly and legitimately prescribed pain medication, so this is an area for special care. When we face a surgery or treatment that does require pain management we need to tell *everyone* ahead of time. Tell your doctors, recovery friends, sponsor, and family members before the surgery. Make a plan so that it's okay for them to check on you when you are using the prescribed medications.

But not all medications are prescribed. We also want to be careful with remedies we buy in the drugstore or at the health food store. A popular tea called kombucha is a true health aid for many people with digestive problems. It's sold in health food stores. But we have to be careful. Kombucha is a fermented beverage. It contains alcohol. That's one example.

A joke I heard recently with an implied warning goes like this: "Be careful with Geritol and NyQuil; there's a reason they come with a shot glass." Yes, those are but two of many over-the-counter medicines that contain a high percentage of alcohol. Read labels, and avoid ingesting even a small percentage of alcohol; even if your drug of choice was marijuana, why risk relapsing over a shot of 50-proof NyQuil?

MENOPAUSE

Women who stay in recovery for a long time will have to face perimenopause and menopause exactly like women who are not in recovery. Yes, real life again. But women in recovery have a few special considerations. For a woman in recovery, menopause can be a time of additional vulnerability.

One of my early sponsors joked about recovering women and menopause saying, "The hormonal swings of menopause can make you feel like you are drunk, and if you have ever been drunk, then you know that the best way to fix that is to have another drink." So we want to be careful as those midlife hormonal changes begin.

Some of the physiological changes for midlife women include loss of muscle mass, changing levels of sex hormones like estrogen and progesterone, and a dropping metabolic rate. Again, these are all pretty normal occurrences, but the consequences and how we feel about them can impact our recovery.

A study from the University of Colorado suggests that over the roughly ten-year period of perimenopause through menopause, about 50 percent of women will gain ten to fifteen pounds because of their lowered metabolic rate. It's safe to say that few women are happy about gaining weight and for most women, both in and out of recovery, that brings feelings of being unattractive, less desirable, and getting old that can jeopardize our sense of well-being.

Menopause raises medication and health questions. Night sweats, insomnia, mood swings, and libido changes all have a physiological basis, but they have emotional and behavioral manifestations, too.

Tabitha Kane, a gynecologist in Albany, New York, confirms, "Most women will see a decrease in libido and they will experience vaginal dryness. The insomnia can be really significant, with resultant irritability. It's a stressful time for any woman. There is a general increase in irritability. Divorces occur."

Concentration and memory can be a problem too, which, for women whose self-image is tied to their professional functioning, is especially hard. "They will take a hit there too," says Dr. Kane. And anxiety can increase. "Some women feel like they're going a little crazy." So with all those factors combined, menopause can significantly affect our relationships and self-image.

Several doctors have confirmed that women who have no history of depression could have more than twice the risk of depression during the menopausal transition. "Yes, this does resolve soon after menopause, but for some women that 'transition' can take a couple of years," according to Dr. Kane.

So how do we sort out our behavior as we are going through menopause? You've heard the jokes:

"Question: What is the difference between a terrorist and a woman in menopause?"

Answer: "You can negotiate with a terrorist."

Yes, it's funny because there's an element of truth.

For a woman in recovery who is trying to be self-aware and mindful of her behavior and her communication—how can she know if her less-than-desirable behavior is evidence of a character defect or the result of declining estrogen?

We have to be mindful at this time because we could either use menopause as an excuse not to take responsibility for our behavior or we could be tempted to try a chemical remedy for our sadness or our anger. We might recall and start to romanticize the ways that wine, marijuana, donuts, or the attention of a new man made us feel better in the past. And yet, we also need to know when professional medical attention and even prescription medications are the right next step.

WHICH BRINGS US TO SEX

For many women it was something in the sexual sphere that got us into recovery. It was either too much or too little, and often it was with the wrong people. Better sex and better attitudes toward sex may be a marker of how far we've come. Pre-recovery, we may have had sex with too many people or the wrong person, or sex was bad because we were numbed out or we didn't have enough sense of self to ask for what we needed.

Even in early recovery we may still have done it with the wrong people—that cute newcomer in our home group or the married guy who was thirteenth-stepping us. But the good news is that as we get better in recovery, our sex life can get better too.

When I was twenty years old I knew so little about sex. When I was twenty-five I thought I knew some things but I still didn't know enough. At thirty I was learning how to give pleasure, but it took almost ten more years to learn how to receive it. And surprisingly, sex does get better with age.

Yes, I always knew that "older" people had sex. When I was thirty-three years old, my seventy-year-old mother, who had been widowed many years, was newly remarried. She told me that she and her second husband, Don, had sex almost every day. I thought, *Good for her*, but I also secretly thought, *How good could sex really be at their ages?* Now I know. And I'm sorry I laughed at the people who told me that sex gets better as you age. I didn't know. But now I do.

At fifty-nine, my sex life is better than I ever imagined. Yes, I wish my skin was smoother and I wish I was firmer, but I now know more about how to give and receive pleasure. Having confidence is part of it—that comes with recovery too—as is learning what works, and being fearless about trying things, and then trying them again.

This is a gift of recovery we don't talk about much in meetings, not even in women-only meetings. But I have learned about my sexual needs and how to meet them. And even that has been a process over years of recovery.

In my pre-recovery and early recovery years all of my character defects applied to my sexual behavior and my sexual sensibility, just as they did to my workplace and social behaviors: I was a people-pleaser, not always honest with others and rarely honest with myself. I didn't know myself well enough to *be* honest.

In those days before recovery, I managed my fear or anxiety with alcohol or other drugs or food, and I was alternately obsessed with my body or wildly out of touch with it—so truly experiencing the sensual didn't have much of a chance.

But I was always an athlete—runner, gymnast, swimmer—so I knew something of the body's mechanics; hence, I learned sex mechanically too, and as a codependent I read every article about how to please men. I knew how to seduce without ever feeling seductive. Yeah, I faked frequently.

In those days before recovery, I managed my fear or anxiety with alcohol or other drugs or food, and I was alternately obsessed with my body or wildly out of touch with it—so truly experiencing the sensual didn't have much of a chance.

But my saving grace was twelve-step recovery, a sponsor who was a nurse, and oddly, Helen Gurley Brown—the longtime editor of *Cosmopolitan* magazine and the author of many books including *Sex and the Single Girl*, which, despite the title, was all about work and careers, not libido. (Helen was married to the movie producer David Brown, who knew the importance of an impressive title.)

Helen's later books were about relationships and aging and sex. In her book *The Late Show*, which she wrote in her sixties, Helen made the point that women over fifty have to decide that they want an orgasm—and then go for it. She got my attention. When I first read that statement I wasn't exactly sure what she meant, but I have since come to understand.

I Am Responsible

It turns out that "going for it" is about self-esteem, self-care, assertiveness, and the best kind of seduction. I can't tell you how glad I am to give up faking it, and in that process I've learned valuable information about my own erotic sensibility. (By erotic sensibility I mean what it takes to get in the mood, which fantasies work for me, and exactly what needs to happen in the, um, athletic sphere.) A woman does need to take responsibility for her orgasm. It may sound a tad "transactional" but it's true. I mean, this too is about being happy, joyous, and free.

Taking responsibility means getting in the mood, using fantasies, erotica, maybe even toys, and it means speaking up. There are countless good books about sexual communication, and with the growing baby boomer demographic, there are many good books on how to keep sex energetic and spirited in a long-term relationship. Women in recovery are passing those books to their friends and they—the books and the friends—are worth it.

AWKWARD OR
UNCOMFORTABLE SEX

Sometimes, and it can happen in new relationships or in longstanding ones, sex gets uncomfortable or awkward. What does a recovering woman do then? Maybe something doesn't work; maybe you can't "perform" or he can't. Or one of you wants something that the other person can't or won't do. Or you both want to try something new and it bombs.

This is, I think, the critical moment when you know whether you are a couple or not. How do you handle sex that doesn't work? Do you laugh? Yes, with each other. Do you cry? Maybe that, too. And then, hopefully you also talk. To each other.

"This is us," I have said. "This is our sex life, not anybody else's; we get to make the rules."

"Yep, this is us," he says.

And then we hold each other.

SURROUNDED BY HELP

All of this means that we need to take care of our bodies. Most of us will need some outside help. It might be from our doctor, gynecologist, therapist, nutritionist, and maybe a massage therapist, coach, or personal trainer.

Our bodies are the vehicles that carry around our minds and our spirits. So as recovery progresses, we need to keep investing in learning about and caring for our physical well-being.

An Important Public Service Announcement: Kegel Exercises

This is information I wish I'd had years ago: Kegel exercises will make your sex life better, with or without a partner. When I learned about Kegels, I swore I'd spread the word to other women, so here goes: To have orgasms and better orgasms you have to have strong pelvic floor muscles. I'm not a doctor, so I won't do an anatomy lesson here but you can look it up. You can Google "Kegel" or ask your doctor or a good friend or your sponsor.

Then do your Kegel exercises. You'll be glad. I promise.

TWIGS FOR CHAPTER TWO:
Physical: Bring the Body

- What new thing are you doing for your healthy body?
  A new food? Exercise technique? What did you love
  as a kid—swimming, dancing, hiking, biking?
  Could you try that now?

- Attend one of the many women's networking nights with
  a focus on women's health. Your local Chamber
  of Commerce or YWCA may be the host.

- Invite a friend and try a new fun kind of exercise: NIA
  (Non-Impact Aerobics or Neuromuscular Integrative
  Action), dance, yoga for round bodies, tap dance or clogging.

Chapter Three

⌒⌇

MENTAL: OUR THINKING GOT US HERE

IN EARLY RECOVERY I READ a little pamphlet called, *Transferring Obsessions*, written by Dr. Judi Hollis. I remember being so mad when my sponsor first gave me that pamphlet and told me to read it, but it had a huge impact on my later recovery and I am grateful to Dr. Hollis to this day.

She was writing to an audience of Overeaters Anonymous members. She talked about what happens when a woman or man in eating disorder recovery begins to let go of that addiction and how, if a higher power is not the replacement, he or she will move on to shopping, decorating, exercising, dating, sex, work, and using alcohol or other drugs. In my OA community, using drugs was frowned on but there were members who still used alcohol, seeing the separation of substances rather than the singularity of addiction.

It was not unlike the way most professionals viewed drug addiction and alcoholism twenty-five years ago. At that time many hospital treatment programs for drug addiction allowed participants to drink alcohol. In some programs people completing their treatment for drug addiction were given a beer bash as the celebration of their ninety days of "clean" time. We are amazed by that today. Maybe someday we'll be amazed by alcohol treatment that allows tobacco use or ice cream parties on Friday nights.

Addiction is one disease with many manifestations. We have a tendency, in recovery, to substitute addictive behaviors and compulsions. It makes sense. Today there are any numbers of things that I can "use"—be it behavior or substance—as a way to "fix my feelings." Conversely, I know that if I can sit still and feel my challenging feelings then I will be much less likely to reach for a substance or behavior to fix me.

Most of us have more than one thing we can use to not feel. You hear it in meetings. Sometimes we hear it spoken about seriously and sometimes as a joke but it's there. The AA member who says he gave up booze but picked up ice cream or the Al-Anon member who comments on her "retail therapy" is talking about this common tendency.

Stay in recovery long enough and you learn that there is truth in those jokes. As recovery progresses we notice that we can get carried away with any number of ways of soothing or numbing our emotions.

We are human beings, and even nonaddicts use food or a new pair of shoes to boost their moods, but those of us who identify as addicts have to be mindful that we can always use a good thing in a bad way to escape our feelings.

Maybe the easiest way to discern whether something is an issue is to apply a few diagnostic questions: Do you feel shame about this? Do you keep this a secret? Does it bother you if someone points out what you are doing? This discernment continues into later recovery. It must.

———

But after many years, we are sitting in the same chairs and saying things that are remarkably similar. The principles of recovery are the same, whatever the substance or behavior.

———

I heard early on that "we will give up our addictive behaviors in the order in which they are killing us." That is why some people enter recovery first for food issues, and others enter for alcohol or other drugs, and yet another person enters to address family or relationship problems. But after many years, we are sitting in the same chairs and saying things that are remarkably similar. The principles of recovery are the same, whatever the substance or behavior.

My entry into recovery brought me face-to-face with transferring addictive activities. Before I went to Alcoholics Anonymous I was confronting my problems with food and relationships. So my first steps toward healing were in Overeaters Anonymous and then in Al-Anon.

Later I began to notice that often when my relationships were rocky, alcohol was a factor. Then I noticed that there was alcohol in my food, too. I told myself that I was "having dessert." But I was "eating" desserts like Irish coffees and ice cream with cups of Kahlua. I asked myself, "How bad could that be?" You didn't see drunks with whipped cream mustaches did you? I always had a spoon in my hand; it was the perfect denial.

So I had to deal with food and relationships *and* alcohol. Under all of it was a messy family history burdened with still more addiction and abuse and shame, but that took years to uncover and to heal.

Alcohol and other drugs may be things of the past, but what about those credit card bills? And what about gambling and sex, and all those shoes? So I work too hard. Is working too hard a *genuine* problem? We have to be willing to keep asking these questions.

That was my experience. As I began to recover from drinking, it got harder to delude myself that certain other behaviors were okay. Without the booze, the hole in my heart began to hurt, and my bargain-basement self-esteem gaped open. I needed soothing. But with what?

As a society, we are familiar with the addictive substances we take into our bodies to change our moods—alcohol and/ or other legal and illegal drugs, nicotine, caffeine, etc. More recently we have begun to recognize the behaviors that we engage in for the same reason—to change our feelings: video gaming, overspending, gambling, sex, and the ever-popular shoe shopping. These are the process addictive behaviors. They are things we do—watching television, overeating, working long hours, starving ourselves, exercising—to change our mood or to avoid growth.

Some things like alcohol and other drugs, nicotine, caffeine, sugar, sometimes salt (who ever eats just one potato chip?) overlap categories as substance addiction or process addiction.

Technology can become a vehicle for process addiction when it's used to avoid emotional discomfort or pain: texting, tweeting, playing games on our phones . . . and on and on and on.

Here's the tricky part, and why I need ongoing discernment involving other people in recovery: The addictive processes are often things that also have good qualities. For example, let's look at exercise.

As we get healthy in recovery we want to get in shape. We start going to the gym or running. But what happens when we miss a day of running or we can't get to the gym? Do we start to feel anxious, angry, and resentful? Some of us exercise for the same reason we used substances: Fix my feelings! I've been there.

And shopping? Who doesn't want to look nice or wear clothes that are becoming? But do we obsess? Spend money we don't have? Wander the mall in a trance? I've done all that, too.

Later in my recovery I had to examine my relationship with money and work. Oh, I had such denial about work. How could something so good be so bad? Wasn't I making up for lost time, finally becoming a productive member of society?

Work, like food, has to be looked at carefully. Putting in long hours may not be the only criterion to use in determining whether or not working is an addiction. We have to look at our motives and at the impact that work has on our health and on the people closest to us.

Some of us in recovery work long hours because we are unhappy at home, or we might work excessively because the workplace is where we can feel total control. Others in recovery may work seven days a week and it's pure joy and all for the good. I think about friends who write or make art or who have small businesses that they love. They pour themselves into their passion and that both reflects and enhances their recovery.

What's under all of it? For me the common denominator under the many manifestations of addiction is a special "cocktail" of shame and fear and feeling "not- good-enough." The shame mantra pushes me toward too many pairs of shoes, or buying expensive gifts simply to impress. I'm still tempted to believe that the right handbag or sweater will fix me. But another woman with that same "not-good-enough" drumbeat in her head won't allow herself anything; she "treats" her shame with deprivation and denial. She might not allow herself to have anything but bargains and secondhand clothes. If you looked at our outsides you'd think we were different but inside we're a matched pair.

We need to keep talking to our sponsors and to women friends about anything that feels uncomfortable, shameful, or that we want to keep secret.

But we keep on. Recovery from our primary behaviors of addiction may have given us our sea legs, but we need to stay vigilant. We need to keep talking to our sponsors and to women friends about anything that feels uncomfortable, shameful, or that we want to keep secret. Those are the signs and hallmarks of addiction. It's your relationship to the substance or behavior—not the substance or behavior itself—that makes the difference.

I ask myself, "Does this behavior stop me from feeling my feelings? Feelings that, if I felt them, would help me to grow?" I know that keeping busy may still be my longest lasting addiction. As my friend Brigid likes to remind me, "Feelings can't hit a moving target."

Can we ever get to the bottom of our addiction? As someone said when I was new in recovery, "If you want to know why you drank, stop drinking and you'll soon find out." It was good advice. When we stop the addictive substance or behavior and we "sit still and feel," the source will reveal itself.

All of this requires discernment, which is defined as judgment, perspicacity, or penetrating insight. (Please note: "judgment" is not always a bad word.)

This is why at a certain point in our recovery we need to find meetings where we can talk about a wide swath of topics. It doesn't help if I am only attending meetings where exclusively the discussion of a particular substance is welcome. By year seven or eight our drunk- or drugalogues have all been told, and may be growing old—but we might be killing ourselves with food, gambling, or sex addiction. We have to shine a light on our patterns—all of our patterns. Something that helps me with this discernment was said by Marion Woodman, Jungian analyst and teacher: "The natural gradient in us is toward growth. Whatever we use repeatedly and compulsively to stop that growth is our particular addiction."

DEPRESSION AND ANXIETY

But what happens when it's not the booze or the blues alone? Compared with men, women with drinking problems are at increased risk for depression, anxiety, low self-esteem, and marital discord. So for women in recovery, coping with clinical depression or another mental illness is frequently an additional serious topic.

This is something that is not talked about often enough in the rooms of recovery even though it is part of long-term recovery and part of getting "out of the woods." As in many fairy tales, the heroine has to go through tests and trials, and in long-term recovery one of our trials may be a period of depression.

We don't talk about it enough because there is a fear of scaring the newcomers, and because there is still some shame about depression and other forms of mental illness. Those of us with longer recovery have to contribute to the erasing of that stigma.

We have a tendency to describe the process of recovery as an upward- and forward-moving trajectory. It goes, "worse, then better, then best, and then until . . ." when? Until our lives are perfect? We know better. If we frame recovery as that always upward-moving escalator, then how can it be that after years of recovery we may start to feel bad?

For many years, there was a dangerous trend in some twelve-step rooms of criticizing people who took antidepressants or antipsychotic medications. Some people with clinical depression or serious mental illness went off their medications to try to be truly abstinent or in the language of twelve-step programs, "clean and sober." Other people drifted away from recovery because they felt their diagnosis made it impossible for them to be part of recovery.

None of us can know for certain what is neurotic and what is neurology. If we suspect that we have a serious issue or if our friends are telling us that they are worried about us, then we need to ask for help without shame; get treatment; and if necessary, take medications as prescribed. That, too, is part of our responsibility to maintaining our ongoing recovery.

It has happened that when someone in recovery goes through a period of depression there are folks in the rooms who will criticize that person's program. Newer members, still on their pink cloud, may whisper about what someone else needs to do. Others might say, "He was not going to enough meetings," or "She didn't really work a program." Maybe not. Many people in long-term recovery have experienced periods of depression. They may have the best programs and they may be ideal students of recovery: going to meetings regularly, being sponsored and sponsoring, and having a seemingly unique or ideal spiritual practice. In fact, there is a belief in certain faiths that some kinds of depression are a "dark night of the soul"—a time when God has moved in extremely close to do deep work, a kind of spiritual surgery. No, that's not fun—but it's also not bad.

Depression can also be a natural consequence of certain situations. It may follow a life event like a divorce or a death, or it may be biologically based. We now know not to criticize people who need to use medications for depression or anxiety. Antidepressants save lives. But there can also be something more to depression in later recovery.

When I went through a depression in my ninth year of recovery, I was told it was "God or Go" time, and that as I was approaching the ten-year mark, it was time to recommit to a higher power. It was also called "dig deep or die" time in old-timer's parlance. The idea was that by the tenth year you pretty much know the program, you have worked the steps and you have reaped significant rewards, but it is time to go to another, deeper layer and that, if you resisted, you'd feel the consequences of your resistance or your inactivity.

In my early recovery I listened often to audiotapes by recovery speakers. I returned to one in particular over and over again because he was so funny and self-deprecating. One of the things that stayed with me about his story was how in his fifth year of recovery he was struck with a depression that left him feeling suicidal.

He talked about trying to look good in meetings and always saying the right recovery things but then, he said, "I'd go home and I'd want to die." Now maybe that doesn't seem like a good thing for a newcomer to hear, but what captured my attention was the sense that this man was telling the truth.

I also knew, because he was telling his story from a later vantage point, that there was more to his story. He had found the way out and I wanted to know what he had learned. There had to be a solution.

His stories, which covered a long period of his recovery, were powerful and helpful. Later, as I too had to face issues of my family or childhood coming to the surface, I knew that while I didn't enjoy it, I was, in a recovery sense, right on time.

It's possible that somewhere between years seven and ten, our underlying family issues will come to the surface with force, especially if there were any sexual abuse issues in the past. According to the National Council on Alcoholism and Drug Dependence (NCADD), "Among drug-using women, 70 percent report having been abused sexually before the age of sixteen."

Whatever has not been talked about or dealt with will eventually come up, and I believe that happens so we can keep healing and growing. Often the symptom of the unresolved gunk in our lives is depression.

No, it's not pretty and it's not fun but when depression is part of recovery, we shouldn't hesitate to get help. We can access resources of all kinds, such as medical, psychological, and spiritual, and we can raise our hands in meetings and talk about it. It won't hurt newcomers to know that all of this is part of a healthy recovering life.

Whatever has not been talked about or dealt with will eventually come up, and I believe that happens so we can keep healing and growing.

ACT. THINK. FEEL.

We have all had those times when despite our hardest work with the tools of recovery and even therapy, we still have some feelings or attitudes that won't shift. It's so frustrating. "I know better, I do. I understand it intellectually at times like that but I still feel mad/sad/resentful/jealous . . . (fill in the blank)." I'll say to my sponsor, "I want the way I feel about the issue to change." Yes, if you were listening to this you'd hear the whine in my voice.

What I want when I feel stuck like that is for my gut to line up with my head and my heart. Those are some of the hardest times in long-term recovery because we are additionally weighed down by the sense that we should know better. We should. I should. I definitely should. (Yes, the whining voice again.)

"Make this shift." I beg my higher power in prayer. Or I say to my therapist, "I want an exorcism." But what do we *do* when there is no magic wand?

I have learned a recipe for those times. It's not magic and it does not work overnight but it does help. It's a three-part therapy that goes like this: first act, then think, and then feel.

Here's an example: In early recovery I struggled with my stepdaughter. She wasn't thrilled that her dad had remarried. I wasn't thrilled that his daughter took him away from me on weekends. I *knew* she wasn't my competition. I *knew* that the better their relationship was, the better it would be for all of us in the long run. I *knew* that I wanted her to have an ever-improving relationship with her father, especially because I'd experienced the lifelong pain of having a less-than-good relationship with my own father. So I didn't want to feel jealous and resentful and petty. But I did.

So after trying pouting, pleading, withdrawing, and basically hurting my marriage, I also tried therapy, and I did an inventory with my sponsor where I focused on parenting and family issues. That helped; I got a much better understanding of where my fears were coming from. I talked—in a sane and reasonable voice—to my husband. It got better, but I still had the feelings, and they were tripping me up.

So I learned the one, two, three of act, think, and feel. I used it like this: First, I started acting, genuine acting, exactly like an actress. I acted like I was happy about their relationship. I acted like I wanted them to have a good time together. I encouraged them to do fun things. I suggested presents I thought she'd like.

I talked to my sponsor every day. With her I could safely vent my feelings and also get a pat on the back for trying.

Then, I started to change my thinking. I began to tell myself that I truthfully wanted their good relationship. I thought about what would make my stepdaughter happy. I thought about her strengths. When I had jealous thoughts, I tried to stop them and replace them with better thoughts. (I used those well-worn cognitive therapy skills of thought stopping by picturing a big red stop sign to shift my attention.)

That was the hardest part. I found that there was some juicy pleasure in staying with the nasty thoughts, so changing my thinking took serious work but it was and is worth it.

Last and finally, I realized that my feelings were actually changing. One day my stepdaughter admired a sweater I was wearing and I thought she would look lovely in it. No, I did not take off my sweater and give it to her. (I'm not a saint and never will be.) But I went back to my favorite store and I bought a second sweater, and I sent it to her. I was happy to do it. That's how I knew the shift had happened. I was genuinely happy to do it. It wasn't about whether she liked me or whether my husband would be impressed with my generosity. I was happy. I was happy to know this attractive young woman who would look terrific in that sweater.

JUST TAKE ME TO THE BEACH

Another helpful thing to learn in recovery is what works for us when we need to process difficult emotions such as anger, sadness, grief, or confusion. Years ago, a relationship expert told me that the best thing you can do in your marriage is tell your partner, well ahead of time, what works best for you when you are having a hard time. She gave the example of a woman who, early in their marriage, told her husband, "When circumstances are glaringly bad for me please don't try to talk to me, but do put me in the car and take me to the beach." They lived in Southern California so that was reasonable. So whenever she had trouble at work, and when the dog was dying, and when her friend was obviously angry, her husband knew that talking would come later—first he needed to take his wife to the beach and let her walk for at least an hour.

I love her idea and I try to be aware of what works for me. It changes over time but my list of "try this first" includes: walking near water, whether the beach, a lake, or a running stream; dancing, either in a class or by simply turning on music and dancing in my living room; and to be near trees, whether in the woods or at a park. It helps me tremendously to lean my body against a tree. Find what works for you and make a list, and tell your partner and close friends so they can remind you.

It seems that at the times when I most need one of these experiences of "emotional first-aid," I'm the first one to forget what will work. Then I'm glad I've told others who can remember.

TWIGS FOR CHAPTER THREE:
Mental: Our Thinking Got Us Here

- What's in your bag of personal growth? Make a list and compare your tools and resources with three recovering friends. Can you try one of their practices?

- Also with close friends: Do a mini inventory of the "subtle" aspects of your addiction. How are you doing in relation to food, television, social media, work, or worry?

- Have you ever been to Al-Anon or OA or NA or DA? Take a friend and visit an open meeting of a different fellowship to expand your perspective of recovery.

Chapter Four

❧

SPIRITUAL:
CAME to UNDERSTAND

MY DAD WAS THERE AT the end of the diving board. He would tread water for hours, watching while I practiced my dives. For years that was our Sunday afternoon ritual. I was four years old when we began. Daddy was there in the deep water, waiting for me. On those Sunday afternoons I believed that if he was there at the end of the board, I could do anything.

He would wait, treading water, off to one side. He would look around and give me the sign that it was okay to dive, and I would stroll to the end of the board, tugging my stretchy lavender swimsuit, and bounce in the air before I dove in.

I would rise to the surface sputtering, and look for his face. He would hesitate a moment to let me right myself. Then he would grab the back of my suit and give me a push toward the side. "Swim to the ladder," he would say. And he would stay out at the end of the board waiting.

I remember the feeling as I paddled to the ladder. The world was perfect. I was in the deep end of the pool; there was no pain and no evil in the world. There was no need or want in my life. I was a perfect, grinning, sunburned, waterlogged four-year-old, in love with the world, herself, and her daddy.

He died when I was eighteen. During the intervening years, life happened.

By the time I was thirteen years old my father was traveling frequently and when we did spend the occasional weekend together we did not speak of personal things. There were no talks about plans or dreams. By then, my addiction had begun.

On a July evening, when he was fifty-six, my father had a stroke and died.

Has it affected me? Of course! To have had that closeness, to have had those timeless moments of being safe and special and then to lose him, well . . . .

It took years of my life, many other relationships, many years of addiction, and many years in recovery for me to reconcile those two men—the daddy who waited in the deep water and the man who left suddenly, without a word, when I was eighteen.

Somewhere inside, that four-year-old still wears her lavender bathing suit. She stands at the end of a diving board and leans forward hoping to hear someone say, "You are so special."

I've learned important lessons from listening to that little girl. I learned that in romantic relationships we get some of that need met, but romance has its own path and, after a while, no one wants to admire us, all day, every day. Another way to meet this need is with an affair. Having an affair is a way a woman's four-year-old self can twirl in her forty-year-old body and hear again, "You are the only one."

In the first five years of recovery I learned healthier solutions. I practiced in the mirror, "Diane, you are special." But all the praise in the world cannot fill a hole that exists in the past or give us the strength to do all that we need to go deeper.

Later I learned to meet this need in a spiritual way. In the rooms I began to meet people who had a connection with their God or higher power that helped them to believe that God smiles on them.

So what is the gift from a father who left when he and I were both too young? It's this: For a long time I resented the missing memories; no father-daughter chats, no drives to college, no adult conversations. But today I believe in a higher power that looks around my life and says, "Hold on a minute. We don't want anyone to get hurt." I have a higher power at the end of my daily diving board that says to me, "Okay now, catch your breath. I'm here."

GET OUT OF GOD'S WAY

One night, when I was in my first few months of recovery, I was in a meeting where a woman shared about a traumatic event the day before in which her young daughter had been badly hurt. The daughter's injuries resulted from a car accident, and the mother was telling the group what happened and how things were going.

The way the woman spoke and what she said made a powerful impression on me, and it made me want recovery. She told the group that on the previous day her young daughter had been hurt when a car jumped the curb near their house and hit the girl. The mother had waited with her daughter until the ambulance came. The mother told the group that she immediately began to pray that her daughter would be okay and asked that God make everything all right.

"But then," she said, "I stopped and changed my prayer. Instead I began to say, 'God, please help me to get out of your way.'"

I was stunned by her words. I was dumfounded that anyone could have the presence of mind or willingness to surrender in the midst of such a frightening situation.

I knew right then that I wanted what she had. I understood that whatever it was that this woman had, it had to have come from participating in this twelve-step program.

That was more than twenty-nine years ago. I still want to have faith that powerful. Her stunning prayer was this: "God, please help me to get out of your way." How do we learn to do that? I think it comes from practicing the Third Step.

STEP THREE

In Step Three, we surrender. "Made a decision to turn our will and our lives over to the care of God *as we understood Him*." That last italicized phrase gives us freedom and flexibility. We don't have to have a Western, Abrahamic God, or the more impersonal God of the Eastern religions—although if we want to, we can. We can have a higher power of our own understanding.

In Step Three, we turn our lives over to something that is bigger than us—something that we don't control. For some of us that might be a pretty traditional God, an anthropomorphized "He," and for others the greater power is an "it" or an idea or a process. The central idea is that we take a leap of faith.

Over the years, whenever taking the Third Step has again become hard for me—and for me Step Three is an "again" process—I often need to reach for my old journals. This is one of the benefits of keeping a journal in recovery and recording the good days and the bad ones. Often in my own journals, I'll find the help I need to remind me that I can rely on Step Three and a higher power.

Because I write almost daily in my journal, the examples are there. I can flip through an old journal and see the problem at work or the relationship difficulty or even practical issues, like times when I struggled with a financial issue, and I can see, in my own handwriting, that I struggled, then I prayed, then I finally turned the issue over, and maybe days or weeks later in that same journal, I see that a solution did arrive. And typically it was a better solution than the one I was insisting on when I was solely relying on myself.

Often in my own journals, I'll find the help I need to remind me that I can rely on Step Three and a higher power.

I need frequent reminders about surrender. It's one of the reasons I still go to meetings. I need repetition. There are some recovery insights that seem so brilliant and obvious that I'm sure "I'll never forget that!" Yet these can turn out to be the exact tidbits of wisdom that I have to hear again and again.

One of the reminders I give myself so often that I keep it on a card on my desk says, "I made a Decision, not a Feeling to turn my will and my life over to God—and that means all of it." That helps me to remember that I don't have to have a big emotional feeling when I surrender.

It also reminds me that I do mean *everything*, even when, in my heart of hearts, I still want to hold something back. Most often, the things I am reluctant to fully and wholly surrender are either related to a relationship ("he/she should like me") or my ego ("please let me be a teeny bit important/special").

THE SPIRITUAL PART OF THE PROGRAM

I love the anecdote we hear in meetings where there's a newcomer who asks about the "spiritual part" of the program and an old timer who replies, "There is no spiritual part—the whole program is spiritual."

Our spiritual growth continues. We look for a higher power in all kinds of places. We find guidance inside and outside the rooms. Some of us come back to the faith of our childhood. Or we begin to shop for a faith community that fits our adult life. We can feel like Goldilocks as we do this: "'This one's too hard; that one's too soft; too strict; this one has bad music, etc., until we find one that is 'just right.'" Recovering people are well-represented in Unitarian Universalist Fellowships and Unity Churches and other ecumenical congregations.

Many of us have found traditional, alternative, and sometimes unorthodox ways to practice the Eleventh Step:

"Sought through prayer and meditation to improve our conscious contact with God as we understood Him." We've been introduced to other religions, other spiritual programs, and a variety of systems of meditation and prayer.

GOD, OF COURSE

The God question, which was there on our first day in recovery, remains. We learned early on that we had to figure out who or what we were turning our lives over to. That desire has led us down some notable paths. Others find that new ways open them to a spirituality that fits their new life. We practice meditation, go on retreats, try sweat lodges, chanting, yoga, and sacred dance. You can find twelve-step women in yoga classes, meditation workshops, and in every kind of church or synagogue and faith community. Many of us meet regularly with a spiritual director.

SPIRITUAL DIRECTION

Though we talk about the Twelve Steps as a spiritual program, we don't often talk about spiritual direction. But outside of meetings, people with many years of recovery may share with each other about spiritual retreats or they might talk about working with a spiritual director or with their pastor or rabbi or a teacher or elder in their faith community.

Our spiritual lives are extraordinarily intimate. In the same way that we don't talk in detail about our sex lives with everyone we are friends with, we typically don't talk about our spiritual lives in detail with a lot of people either.

Don Bisson, a spiritual director from Rhinebeck, New York, told me that the intimacy we experience with God requires the same skills as the intimacy we experience with another person. Intimacy with another human being *is* intimacy with God—there is no difference.

A spiritual director can be someone who is wiser than us on spiritual matters whom we can talk to about spirituality on an intimate basis. A spiritual director is not a sponsor and not a therapist, and he or she may or may not be a member of the clergy or part of a religious body.

Over the years I have worked with three different spiritual directors. One was a Catholic nun, one a former Methodist minister, and one an unusually compassionate and spiritual woman who had training in spiritual direction. All had some experience with the Twelve Steps and recovery programs.

There are spiritual directors in every faith community—it's not necessarily a Christian thing. And it's not purely a recovery thing. Most faith communities offer spiritual direction for anyone in their congregations. It can be welcome help and an adjunctive support to people in recovery.

There are spiritual directors who work with people who are atheist or agnostic. Some people who don't believe in a God also want to have more spirituality in their lives or they want to connect to something bigger than themselves. Those who consider themselves humanists may choose nature or science or beauty as a higher power, and a spiritual director might help them as well.

During those times in my life when I could not connect to a God or a higher power, I was always able to get peace by going to the beach. There was no question for me, when looking at the ocean, that it was bigger and more powerful than me. My spiritual director helped me to find rituals that embraced the ocean as my higher power. To this day when I go to the beach—in Florida or California or my favorite, the Coast Guard Beach on Cape Cod—I plan time for myself to be alone there, and I use a stick to write the names of people I love or people I am struggling with in the sand near the water's edge. Then I watch as the ocean takes them away into its bigness.

In a way, a spiritual director is a bit like a couples' counselor. If I am trying to have a genuine relationship with a higher power then anything that might come up in a human relationship will come up in this relationship as well. I tend to have similar questions and expectations. It might be about trust, honesty, or self-revelation.

My spiritual director asks me, "Are you talking to Him?" and "Are you listening to Him?" She reminds me that I can express all of my feelings—even anger—when I am in a genuine relationship with my higher power.

Not long ago I found myself confused about forgiveness. Certainly, forgiveness is an important value in a good spiritual life, and certainly people in recovery are often (but not always) the recipients of forgiveness when we make amends for harms we have caused. So I thought of myself as a forgiving person. I had worked through some forgiveness challenges over the course of my recovery and healing from childhood abuse.

But a current situation had me stumped. A woman I'd known for some time—I'll call her Mary—had gossiped about me. The awful things she said got back to me and I was hurt and mad. After talking with my sponsor I went to speak to Mary. I was nervous but I said that I knew what she had done, and she apologized. We talked about our feelings and our fears and it felt like one of those intense recovery moments when you do the right thing and the right thing happens as a result.

But then, a month later, I heard that Mary was still gossiping about me, and that she had shared some of the personal information I had shared with her when we had our "heart-to-heart" talk. I decided that rather than confronting her again I'd keep some distance.

I wondered if I was being unforgiving. A conversation with my spiritual director helped. She said, "Forgiveness does not create a relationship." She added, "You can forgive her and you can have empathy for her brokenness, but it's also self-caring to stop offering her information that she can use as gossip." Having boundaries, my spiritual director said, was part of forgiveness.

Spiritual directors can also help us learn about and try new spiritual practices as well. Like I need to keep mixing it up in my physical fitness realm—keeping a changing mix of walking and yoga or Pilates, sometimes adding in Zumba or a cardio-fitness class—I sometimes need to try new things with my spiritual practices as well. The past month I've been working with the Examen—a form of prayer taught by Saint Ignatius to his followers. In the Examen, he taught them to spend a period of reflection each evening in which they were to ask God to show them the good and bad of their day and they were always told to pay attention to where they had felt the presence of God in their day. That ancient practice was handed down to The Oxford Groups and became the basis of our Tenth Step daily inventory.

MANTRAS, MIRACLES, AND MIXING IT UP

I sense that women in long-term recovery may be disproportionately represented in alternative forms of worship and in New Age practices. We pray, meditate, chant, and participate in rituals. We show up at solstice celebrations and we try Native American practices. We mix it up by going to church and to Buddhist meditation groups and to trance dance workshops. We've taken many of the roads less traveled on our way out of the woods.

An early part of my recovery included working with *A Course in Miracles*. I was in the first few months of recovery and pretty raw; a relationship was ending and I took off to California to visit my older sister. I didn't tell her much about what was going on. I feared her disapproval. She was "the good one" in our family.

We've taken many of the roads less traveled on our way out of the woods.

My sister, a former elementary school teacher, was working as the Director of Faith Education at a Methodist Church. I was enjoying this break at her house by taking long walks on the beach in the morning, reading in the afternoon, and then cooking for her family each night. I didn't talk about what was going on at home and my sister wisely didn't ask.

One night when my sister came home from work, I perfunctorily asked about her day and what was new at work. "Well," she said, "There's a woman at the church starting a group on how to make miracles." My sister thought it was kind of odd and not very interesting, but something in me leapt. Maybe I knew that I needed some miracle or maybe I knew that my baby steps into twelve-step recovery were the start of my miracle, but I asked for more. "I'll bring you her flyer," my sister said, and the next day she brought home the flyer describing an *Introduction to the Course in Miracles*. I remember thinking, "Maybe this will help me too." And it did.

When I got back to Baltimore I found a local group and jumped in. More a philosophy than a religion, the course teaches about love and forgiveness. I found that there were people in twelve-step recovery in this course. I began to connect spiritual growth with healing my disease of addiction.

THE SOUNDS OF SILENCE

Perhaps a central part of any of these spiritual practices is that we learn to be comfortable in silence. We learn that we can access a higher power or our own inner wisdom by being silent sometime during our day.

One of my early spiritual directors told me this: "God's voice is subtle. Each day in prayer, look for the thing that struck you that day—maybe an impulse or a thought or an image." She told me that by being quiet in some part of my day, I could train myself to see and sense the subtle. And by doing that I was hearing a higher power or my own best, wise self.

The lesson of silence was reinforced in a yoga class I attended. The teacher would remind us that slowing the body had many benefits and would say to us, "When the mind and body are still—and quiet—wisdom effortlessly reveals itself."

WE HAVE GOOD HABITS

Years ago I thought that people who had many years of recovery must have been following all the right practices all of the time for as long as they'd been in recovery. But they haven't, and we don't need to, either. We need to do enough right, enough of the time, to establish good recovery habits. The trouble is no one, not even those who have long-term recovery, knows exactly what those "right practices" are. So we keep doing *all* of it—the program and the fellowship parts of our recovery.

The other helpful things that people in long-term recovery have are stories. We have our own stories yes, but, even better, we have other people's stories too. If you go to meetings for years, you accumulate stories. So when times are hard I can lean into others' stories. I can recall what they said about the time they prayed, the time they yelled at God, the time a prayer was answered in a miraculous way; they let go of what they wanted and got something so much better instead.

When I hear folks with long-term recovery talk, what impresses me most is their willingness. I hear their willingness to use the tools of recovery; their willingness to admit when they are wrong; and their willingness to say, "I don't know. You may be right."

Acceptance requires willingness, and forgiveness is one benefit of willingness.

Our friends with strong recoveries can show us what it looks like to have a willingness to believe in a higher power and a willingness to surrender one's life and will to that higher power. Yes, there is still that "giving-up and taking back thing," and no one does this perfectly, but I admire the willingness of people in recovery who do more than concede or give up or go along with what is happening. Instead, they practice a kind of active and, well, willing, willingness.

Willingness is more than acquiescing, more than gravity. An apple falling from a tree may or may not be willing. But a person who tries skydiving, bungee jumping, or slipping into the deep end of the swimming pool for the first time is showing willingness. Acceptance requires willingness, and forgiveness is one benefit of willingness.

And, as we've been told over the years, you only need a little bit of willingness to make a shift. One of my favorite sayings about willingness is "Willingness is a grace and a softening. It is leaving the door slightly ajar." And willingness is freedom.

NEGATIVE CAPABILITY

The poet John Keats first used the term "negative capability" to describe the state and the process of being with the unknown. He valued this ability in writers and thinkers, describing negative capability like this: "It is when a man is capable of being in uncertainties, mysteries, doubts, without any irritable reaching after facts and reason."

I think this is also something that we strive for in recovery and perhaps use less elegant language to describe. Being comfortable in the unknown, and accepting doubt, is not far from "Living life on life's terms."

FACING FEAR

We learn early in recovery that fear is the root of our character defects. We also know—before we even read any recovery literature—that fear was underneath much of our addiction. We were afraid of people, of social activities, of responsibilities and maybe, sadly, afraid of our own dreams.

Therefore, facing and managing fear is a huge part of our recovery. It continues as long as we are recovering. What changes as we go further into a recovered life is that we recognize our fears faster, we name them correctly, and we have strategies that we use to manage them.

But here's the tricky part in long-term recovery: We have also learned to trust our gut. We have been learning to pay attention to our intuition and the "still small voice" inside. Often that small voice is our higher power trying to reach us. So when discomfort about a task or an effort is present, it takes some practiced discernment to know: Is this our inner wisdom cluing us in and saying, "Walk away"? Or is it fear dressed up in some new way? It's not easy to tell.

This is also why we still have sponsors and twelve-step friends, and it's why we practice prayer and meditation. It's why we make sitting still a habit. When we get as quiet as we can get and ask our higher power to speak to us, we often sense a subtle shift and then we have a better idea if the discomfort is wisdom, or simply fear.

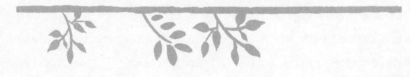

TWIGS FOR CHAPTER FOUR:
Spiritual: Came to Understand

- Can you describe your spiritual practices and habits?

- Consider exploring a spiritual practice that's new to you. Maybe contemplative prayer, meditation, or chanting.

- Perhaps with a friend, explore and visit two spiritual/ faith communities that you've wondered about: A different church, Unity fellowship, meditation sangha group, contemplative prayer, liturgical dance, etc.

Chapter Five

MAKING MEETINGS WORK

WHILE THE TWELVE STEPS ARE the spiritual and philosophical center of twelve-step recovery, going to meetings is the educational and practical center of how we develop a program of recovery and connect with other recovering people.

So as we advance in years of recovery the question arises: How many meetings should you attend? In early recovery there is an abundance of good advice. People who are brand new are advised to do "ninety in ninety"—which means going to ninety meetings over the course of ninety days or three months. Some people do that by going to one meeting every day for three months or sometimes going to two in a day if they need to get enough meetings to make a total of ninety.

So What's Your Number?

I have heard the suggestion that you should go to the same number of meetings each week as the number of days you used your drug or behavior of choice during your active addiction. When some people have balked at attending meetings on holidays or in bad weather someone might say, "If I would have gone out in my active addiction on this day then I can go out in my recovery as well."

But later, in our "out of the woods" phase of recovery, how many meetings should we attend to keep a good recovery program going? Regular meeting attendance is the smartest and safest way to go, but I have known people with more than twenty years of recovery who attend three meetings a week and others who attend only one meeting each week. Some women attend even less frequently when their lives are busy, but they make sure to stay in close contact with recovery friends until they get back to regular meetings.

Because many of us do keep exploring new areas of growth we may have added more than one kind of twelve-step group over the course of our recovery. In my area of upstate New York some people refer to themselves as "double winners" because they are members of two different twelve-step fellowships.

The number and the kinds of groups we attend will depend on our needs at the time and perhaps on what issues are most pressing. A woman whose child is struggling with addiction may need to attend twelve-step fellowships that are specifically for family members more than any other fellowship at that time.

Similarly, someone who is coming face-to-face with her own spending or shopping might want to make a regular commitment to Debtors Anonymous (DA) and decrease her attendance at OA or Al-Anon. If something in our lives has triggered an exacerbation of early abuse issues or family-of-origin issues we may want to make a concentration in Adult Children of Alcoholics (ACOA) or Codependents Anonymous (CoDA), with or without counseling, such as, for example, an abuse or incest survivors group.

Some women attend one kind of meeting each week over the course of a month. They might go to AA one week, Al-Anon the next, and OA the next, and then circle around again.

Despite my early hopes about how recovery worked, I had big plans to "graduate" in a couple of years, I now know that recovery is ongoing and sometimes my path is a spiral. We may touch on the same issues again over the years but we are at a new place and hopefully learn faster each time we make a new circuit. We make meeting attendance an important part of life, but we also "have a life."

THE CHATHAM, MASSACHUSETTS WOMEN'S GROUP

While writing this book I had the wonderful experience of visiting the Thursday morning women's meeting on Cape Cod. I'd heard about the meeting but since it's on a weekday I'd never attended. But during my writing weeks on the Cape, I found the Thursday Women's Step Meeting.

This particular meeting has been in existence for more than thirty years, so it's not the oldest meeting, but what is unique is that among the sixty regular members, more than one-third have more than twenty years of recovery. A dozen of the regulars have thirty or forty years in recovery. So I knew this was a place to ask my questions.

When I asked, "Why do you still go to meetings?" I heard, "Because it would be selfish not to—I remember the women who were here when I came in. I want to be that for someone else." And I heard, "People do relapse no matter how many years they have," and this was always followed by a story about someone with many years who had recently relapsed. I also heard from Ellen who recently celebrated twenty-nine years, "I go to two meetings a week now: a regular step meeting so that I keep growing and I go to an open discussion meeting so that I can stay open to helping others."

JUST LIKE TAKING A DAILY VITAMIN

Someone asked me how, in early recovery, when I was filled with fear and anxiety, I had been able to let go of my addiction to alcohol and food. I thought about that question and answered, "Well, I went to a meeting every day, and I talked about what was going on almost every day, and I called someone—or several people—in the program every day." What I did in my first three and five and ten years was to use the program and the tools. So now, many years later, when I have to think through some fear, I sometimes think, *So why don't I do now what I used to do then?* What if I were to go to more meetings? Talk about what's going on . . . call someone in the program . . . every day, just like taking a vitamin? What helped me then can help me again.

*What I did in my first three and five and ten years
was to use the program and the tools.*

WHEN YOUR MEETINGS
HAVE TO CHANGE

When I was in my twelfth year of recovery—at about that same point of recovery as my friend Miriam was when she made me the "stages" quilt with the "messy but colorful" square—I fell in love with a man who lived six hours away from me. I lived in Baltimore, Maryland and he lived in Glens Falls, New York.

Because I had a solid base of recovery I did know better than to immediately hire a moving van and take off, as had been the possibility in years one or two of recovery; but this was a good man and a good relationship.

We dated long distance for a year. We met each other's friends. We stayed in each other's homes. We talked about tough things like God and money and sex and our family-of-origin experiences and the resulting effect on our lives. We each had a sponsor and a therapist and after a year everyone agreed: this was a good thing. But his work was tied to his community and as I was ready to make a career change, I moved to upstate New York.

I had good recovery habits. I was going to three or four meetings a week in Baltimore. My friends at those meetings knew my history and I knew theirs. I understood what they were trying to change and they knew what I was trying to accept. We spoke in shorthand. For example, when Dave the Dentist said, "So I called the plumber," we all laughed. Or when "Garden Mary" talked about her daughter we understood that she was talking about a beloved child who died years before. It also happened that many people in my Baltimore home group were also in therapy and Al-Anon or ACOA, so no one cringed when someone talked about their "issues" or "processing their feelings" or doing "anger work."

After my first week in my new community I sought out meetings, and the first surprise was that there were so few. I was used to being able to choose from five to seven on any given day and there was always a meeting that I could walk to. Now, in a more rural area, there were only three meetings every week.

But I got directions and I went. I knew the rules: "Try six meetings." And "Each meeting has a personality." But I was unprepared for the culture shock. In the first new meeting forty-five minutes from my home, I listened through the familiar readings and introductions, and then raised my hand to speak. I got stares. It turned out that it was considered arrogant to volunteer. Humility was expressed in waiting to be called on.

When the chairperson acknowledged me I said I was new and began to describe some of my feelings about having a new home and a new job in a new city and all the displacement and loss, exhilaration and grief I was experiencing. I had spoken for a few minutes when a man across from me slapped his hand down on the table and said, "Stop whining, you're not unemployed and you have a roof over your head." I gulped, looked around and sized up the crowd. There were mostly men, and by the looks of things, plenty of poverty. Maybe I had been oblivious; how could I talk about the "issues" that I was struggling with?

It took a long time to find meetings that felt a little more familiar, and I had to drive almost an hour to another city to participate in them. That was hard.

Then I had to make myself known, and learn the new norms. Any pink that was left in my pink cloud had faded to mud. I would skip a week and then go back to another meeting. I'd force myself to go to the same meetings several times. It felt grim and perfunctory. I volunteered for service, raising my hand and speaking to the group leaders but didn't get picked. That hurt too. All the while I kept calling my old recovery friends back in Baltimore and yes, I did whine.

Thankfully the recovery habits I'd developed in my first dozen years, and my fear of relapse, kept me trying. It was not easy; it was not fun and I worried that I'd never connect to recovery again in the way that I had in Baltimore.

It took more than a year to feel like I was part of recovery again, and almost three years to truly be part of a home group in my new upstate New York recovery community.

When I chair meetings these days I often say that one of the hardest things I faced in recovery was moving to a new community. When I meet people who are new to Albany, my current hometown, I offer a hearty welcome and I make sure to introduce them around. I also tell them that it's okay to hate this new place, but please keep coming to meetings and find the rest of us who made moves like this and who understand what this particular discomfort in the middle of recovery feels like.

WHO'S ON YOUR TEAM?

While I was visiting Cape Cod I went to have a pedicure. When the woman doing my pedicure asked why I was on the Cape I took a breath and said, "I'm writing a book." "What's it about?" she asked. "Well," I said, taking another breath, "it's about women in twelve-step recovery." And I paused, not sure what would happen next. "Are you in recovery?" she asked. And I nodded. Then she said, "I am, too, ten years." We had a lively conversation.

She explained further, "You need seven people in recovery who you know well enough—and who know you well enough—so that you can call them any time."

When I asked her about sponsorship she told me about her sponsor's advice. "You need to have your own softball team," she was told. "You need seven people who you can call in as needed; seven women who are your team." She explained further, "You need seven people in recovery who you know well enough—and who know you well enough—so that you can call them any time." I had never heard that advice before and I thought it was terrific.

I immediately and discreetly started counting on my fingers. Yep, I have seven. So that's another mini-guideline for ongoing recovery. Do you have seven women who you know well enough to call anytime? That means seven women who are watching you recover as you are watching them. And of course to get and keep those seven you have to be in meetings on a regular basis to keep recruiting for your team.

That original seven won't be the same seven a few years from now. Life happens, schedules change, we get new jobs, fall in love, and sometimes we move to a new town. So to make sure you have a strong roster on your softball team you want to be in those rooms watching and listening like a good scout.

BOREDOM

"I am so sick of recovery," my friend Tammy says on my voicemail. She is calling to vent. Tammy has had terrific recovery for almost twenty years. I listen to her long message while I unpack my lunch at my desk, "I'm so torn" she goes on. "I know my recovery got me this life that I have—career, husband, kids who are doing so well—but meetings are boring and I fight with myself to get there once a week."

Seems like heresy doesn't it? Things we are not supposed to say. But I have been there too; in fact I come and go from the "bored with meetings" place. What does that mean?

In early recovery, if we voiced a sentiment of boredom with recovery we'd bring down the wrath of sponsors and other recovering people. We'd be admonished, "You are in danger; your recovery is at risk." The suggestions would include, do more service, work the steps, get some humility, and try some new meetings. That last suggestion is one that still works when boredom hits in later years.

Women in long-term recovery do get bored sometimes. We need to be able, like Tammy, to safely say that out loud.

No, maybe we don't want to say that around the newcomers, and not to the people we sponsor if they have less than ten years. But it is true: sometimes we get bored or tired or cranky about recovery. But with long-term recovery, as I've discussed, comes discernment—the knowledge of when, how much, and with whom to share what. Newcomers need our experience, strength, and (most of all) hope. It's best to save sharing what could be interpreted as complaining with others who will understand.

Many women with longer recovery feel bad about this, and there are people in recovery who will try to shame women who are going through this stage. But there is no need for shame, blame, or panic; it is just that, another stage of recovery. The truth is that this stage of recovery, with its blessings and opportunities, also involves struggles and ambivalence that are not often spoken of openly.

But What's Enough?

So how do you know what's enough? If or when it's okay to take a break? In early recovery we'd track down local meetings when we traveled on business or on a family vacation. Our families learned that we could only go out for ice cream after Mom went to her meeting. But now, maybe we go a week with no meeting, or upon return from vacation we jokingly tell our home group that maybe eight days was one day too long.

Is there a time to go back to two or three meetings a week? If we have something tough going on at work or home, or a time of big emotional growth—then we will want extra meetings and that may be the time to take a service commitment in a meeting to ensure that we get there on a regular basis.

I have found and recommended to others that when we make a geographical change—moving to a new city or town—that is an excellent time to go back to the old standard of "ninety in ninety." That commitment forces us to remake our meeting habit and it gets us connected to recovering people in the new community. Ninety days assures that we'll see and be seen, and we'll have time to hear enough new people to select a new sponsor if needed.

Probably the safest guideline is a minimum of one or two meetings a week and preferably in a home group so that we are known, seen, and connecting with our recovery friends and peers.

Is there a correct number of meetings? Probably the safest guideline is a minimum of one or two meetings a week and preferably in a home group so that we are known, seen, and connecting with our recovery friends and peers. A home group gives us a safe place to talk about everything that happens in our lives. Some of us still go to three meetings a week while others go once a week and add some retreats or workshops to their meeting schedule.

It's also likely after ten or twenty years that we'll have recovering friends who we see outside of meetings. So maybe we are also having lunch or dinner once a week with one or more other recovering women. We need to be able to speak the language of the heart and the language of personal growth.

So those cups of coffee can have the quality of a meeting as well. What we most need is a place where and people with whom we can share everything. No secrets. No shame. No pretending.

For some women, meetings take place in new ways. Yes, that's officially unofficial, but we know it happens. Recovering women meet for lunch or dinner or take weekly walks together and keep working their program in those less formal settings. While these gatherings lack a preamble or a prayer, they are conversations that offer community with other recovering women and are a complement to regular meetings.

A New Meeting, a New Home Group, a New Sponsor, Oh My!

When I fell in love with that man from New York in my twelfth year, I had to make two huge changes: I had gained a new relationship and lost the daily presence of my Baltimore home group and the people who knew me so well. I was challenged with making new friends who didn't use in a new recovery community. It wasn't easy.

Here's what I'd do differently if I were moving to a new city today:

- I'd be quicker to realize that in many ways, I'd be a newcomer again.

- I'd try to expect there to be bumps and uncomfortable feelings exactly like in the first chronological year of recovery. (It could even be a tad more uncomfortable because I'd have felt known and understood for a long time in my home group and home-city.) Think about it; in a new place, no one knows your story or your jokes or your references.

It used to be that you'd laugh and your old home group would laugh whenever you'd say, ". . . and then I sold the car . . ." but these new people don't laugh. They don't know your joke—or you. And you don't know them.

Also, if you move a long distance you may find that recovery is done differently in the new place. The meetings are ninety minutes or fifty-nine minutes and sponsees are called pigeons or babies and you have to be called on to share in meetings—raising your hand is frowned on—or vice versa. It's hard not to call your old sponsor and complain about how they do it all wrong.

You may want a local sponsor. Again, like a beginner you have to go through the uncomfortable experience of asking a stranger to be your sponsor—and then actually calling her! It is too tempting to call back to the old hometown and former sponsor. That new sponsor will help you connect to meetings, and that's important to keeping your recovery alive in a new place. Of course we need to keep close to our program literature and continue working the steps, but even those are easier when we are part of a recovery community. When we move to new cities or towns in recovery it can be too easy to drift away.

There is also the paradox—one of many in recovery—

that comes after ten or more years: There is much less pain and crisis in our lives. Those are good things. But in the early days it was pain and crisis that kept us attending meetings on a regular basis. Many of us were learning from scratch how to live, and that assured daily contact with sponsors and other program folks.

So while we have less pain, or maybe better skills to handle it in later recovery, we don't have that same urgent push to stay connected. But that's the danger. Another saying applies here, "People who don't go to meetings don't find out what happens to people who don't go to meetings."

Many of us were learning from scratch how to live, and that assured daily contact with sponsors and other program folks.

We want to keep the good recovery that brought the good geographic changes into our lives, so we have to practice the humility of being both an old timer and a newcomer again.

TWIGS FOR CHAPTER FIVE:
Making Meetings Work

- Do you have a regular meeting schedule? Jump-start yours again by attending "thirty in thirty," or even "ten in ten."

- Do you always attend the same meetings? Challenge a friend and try four new meetings in six weeks.

- If business or pleasure takes you out of town, go online and find a meeting near where you'll be staying. Show up early, raise your hand to speak, and after the meeting, ask about the best local restaurants.

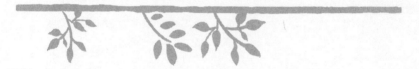

Chapter Six

❧

LOVE and ROMANCE LATER

I HAVE ALWAYS LOVED RECOVERY slogans. I like the old ones the most because they give a sense of what recovery was like in the early days. One of my favorites from the 1930s is "Under every skirt's a slip." I laugh every time I read it and it makes me pause to remember that Alcoholics Anonymous was a de facto men's program in its earliest days. They warned each other about the ways that women could jeopardize recovery. But the reference to "slips" makes me smile too. Today most of us know Spanx better than slips, but the point is still clear: Relationships and love affairs are tricky territory for recovering people.

In early recovery the rules are pretty clear. (Not that we follow them, necessarily.) Those funny stories often begin with, "They told me in my first year that I was not to date, but . . ." And that "but" and that ellipsis are always the prelude to a heartbreakingly funny story. Someone will share about the relationship gone awry, about some romantic undertaking with another newcomer or how they were snookered by an old timer bent on thirteenth-stepping newcomers.

The rules are there for a reason, and we did better when we followed the rule to not date or maybe not even get divorced in that first crucial year.

Some of us came into recovery not wanting any romance. Some of us came in gun-shy and guy-shy. Some women had given up relationships, so after a couple of years of recovery they had to be coaxed into dating. Others among us had to learn the difference between dating and wedding planning. Three dates doesn't mean you are engaged.

In recovery some of us do remarry; some decide never to marry, and some of us stay with the same person we were with when we got into recovery. Those folks often have to do the heavy lifting of marriage counseling. Some of us decide to have serial—but intact and decent—relationships. We take responsibility for the sex, the sexuality, and the money, those tricky issues that often bog us down in romantic relationships.

Sometimes people discover that they were using addiction to cope with a different sexual orientation, and they then have the pain and the joy of coming out in recovery. They also have to learn how to date. In our home groups we held each other's hands and passed the tissues. We endured the heartbreak. And broken hearts are harder to handle when you are not using because you feel everything more intensely.

Sometimes, especially as our recovery continues, we feel an additional layer of pain and shame because we were so sure that we'd be wiser in recovery. We felt the frustration of believing that surely, after all the recovery work we had done, we could make a relationship or a marriage work *this* time. Sometimes we learn that no matter how committed we are, that one person can't make a relationship work.

By the time we have ten or more years we have integrated our recovery values deeply enough that we can recognize a decent person, and we don't require him or her to come wrapped in a twelve-step package.

So what are the rules for love and romance for a woman who has more than ten years of recovery? Well, we know that some of the things we swore by earlier in our recovery aren't necessarily true now. Our partners don't have to be people who are also in twelve-step recovery.

By the time we have ten or more years we have integrated our recovery values deeply enough that we can recognize a decent person, and we don't require him or her to come wrapped in a twelve-step package.

Yes, it helps if our partners have some understanding of what that's all about, and it helps if they are committed to some kind of personal or spiritual growth for themselves. But it's no longer true, as I once imagined, that I could only be with a man who shared my commitment to recovery.

It's even possible that there are some good men and women out there who don't have many life issues to recover from. What we do need though is a partner who understands that recovery is important to us.

Another change is that we don't all have the same rules for our households that we might have had early on. Some of us are as strict as we were in our first ninety days: We don't go to bars or parties where there will be liquor; we don't keep alcohol or other drugs or trigger foods in our homes. Other recovering people have beer in the fridge for their in-laws and it's truly no big deal, while some of us will never serve liquor, not even at our own daughters' weddings.

It turns out, we are delighted to learn, that in this dating and relationship area, we are like other women. We're a little older and we wonder where all the good ones went. Some of us date younger men, some come into (or come out to) our true sexual orientation and find a female partner of whom we ask and to whom we offer the same respect and commitment.

We also discover that when we begin to date again or start a new marriage, women's meetings are gold. It's rewarding to have other recovering women with whom to discuss sex and thighs and hair loss and jealousy and to laugh and cry about it all.

I love relationship books. I absolutely love them. I often think that I should be better at relationships given how many books I read, but maybe it's more like the opposite. Because I see my own struggles, I am fascinated by what psychology and medicine and theology and even astrology have to say about how to find, make, keep, and grow in a loving relationship.

This week I'm reading an old favorite, *Change Your Mindset Not Your Man*, by Sally Watkins, MSW. One of her main points is that most women have relationship troubles because we lie to ourselves. The man is bad? Well, she asks, what red flag did you choose to ignore? If the man is really bad and you are still there, then this is all about you, according to Sally. Yeah, that is hard to hear, but sometimes those buckets of cold water are shockingly refreshing.

How Much Together? How Much Apart?

Another key issue in relationships is balancing intimacy and autonomy, that is, how to identify the midpoint between caring and self-sacrifice. How do I love and care for my partner and not lose myself? This is the challenge. It's about finding balance.

In recovery many of us have the opportunity to do marriage differently. I was saying to a friend that I wished I had more time alone at home. My husband is a teacher and when he is off in the summer, I miss my mornings alone in the house. My friend's husband travels for work and so she has more than enough alone time, but she misses those daily dinners they shared when his previous job brought him home every night.

It is true that the grass is always greener, but it's also true that we each have a preference for how much autonomy and how much dependency we like. It's almost as if we each have a set point. (That's also why many of us couldn't be married to someone else's spouse, no matter how green their grass looks from our window!)

I remember in early recovery a therapist explaining to me that the hardest work a couple has to do is learn their preferences, and then negotiate the middle. I knew that I was a "distancer," always pushing away, making space, and when I was in the midst of addiction I was the one who left. What I learned was that my distancing simply hid my own need for dependence. When a new guy stayed away then I got to feel that yucky, dependent, needy, caring feeling. I could be the distancer until a man took more distance than I was comfortable "letting" him have, then I would tiptoe back toward coupledom and closeness.

It was similar for my friend who says she likes to be close and have plenty of time together. When her husband was laid off for eight months and was waiting at the door each night, she took longer and longer to get home from work each day.

That's part of what we get to do when we are in recovery a long time; we learn about ourselves and we learn what is underneath our first reactions. A good relationship needs to allow for intimacy and autonomy for both partners. In the course of my recovery, I have erred on both sides. Too much him and not enough me, and then in another relationship I kept too much distance. It takes sorting.

I have come to believe that when we say of any other person's behavior, "Can you imagine?" that in fact we actually can. And that's what upsets us. We each have it in us to be dependent and also to want to run away. Psychologists talk about "reaction formation" in which we do the exact opposite of what we want or fear. My fear of being dependent, or of having someone be dependent on me, is likely some of the fuel in my "independence" and distancing.

The gift of long recovery is learning about ourselves. And then, if we have the courage to face what we learn, we can create healthy relationships with our partners.

MARRIAGE IS AN ART

Marriage is a creative act. The materials are expensive, there is an audience, and there is no net. The legality adds a risk factor. Perhaps marriage is a kind of performance art created in front of a live audience. Or maybe it's installation art that is bizarrely conceptual and wildly improvisational.

A spiritual director who I talked with about relationships told me that "the purpose of marriage is to find the right person to force you to individuate. The goal of marriage is not happiness but individuation."

Marriage is a creative act. The materials are expensive, there is an audience, and there is no net.

I once watched a well-done video of cellist Yo-Yo Ma and choreographer Mark Morrison working together on Bach's cello suites. It struck me that Yo-Yo Ma had to find an artist of his caliber with whom to collaborate on this creation. Watching him with Morrison I could see this had to be an undertaking between two artists who had the same degree of skill, expertise, giftedness, and ego to make an effective collaboration.

Maybe this is also true in marriage. Each partner has to have confidence in him- or herself, a belief in his or her own creativity, health, passion, ability, intelligence, and the ego strength to both hold his or her ground and cede the ground as needed. "Collaboration" may be a better word in relationships than "partnership." Partnership suggests each puts some part of themselves aside in order to make the relationship work, but collaboration requires strength and humility, the ability to suggest, to insist but also to step aside and be taught without loss of face or ego.

You Have to Take All of It

A friend of mine told me an extremely helpful piece of advice that her sponsor gave her when she was thinking about marrying the man with whom she had been living. Her sponsor told her to get quiet and "make a list of all the things that upset you, annoy you, and that you don't like about him." Then carefully look at that list and ask yourself, "Can I accept each item on that list?" If you can, then you can marry him because those will not change.

But What about Adultery?

"If my husband ever . . . ." With each round of celebrity infidelity we engage in the age-old game of "If my husband ever . . . ." At fifty-nine, I've played this many times at lunch tables and water coolers and while sitting on the floor in a girlfriend's living room. But at fifty-nine I've also taken enough early morning phone calls from some of those same friends to know that even if you think you know what you'd do if you discovered a partner's infidelity, you don't.

Some leave at once, some never leave, some forgive, some don't. Sometimes, the ones who forgive stay, but sometimes leaving turns out to be the route to forgiveness. Most chilling,

I think, are those who never leave, never separate, and never forgive. They keep up appearances. Maybe they are even envied by others for their "perfect" marriages, which are glued together with hatred and spite.

The agony of infidelity does not discriminate. There is enough to go around. I've played all the parts: scorned wife, secret lover, other woman, and the friend who knew. There are no winners.

IN ALL OUR AFFAIRS

The sad fact is that sometimes the "affairs" are literally, "affairs." In the general population it's reported that upward of 60 percent of married women have had an affair and that maybe 70 percent of women have had a relationship with a married man.

I can't throw stones. In my first year of recovery I "fell in love" with a man in my recovery group who was married. We had an affair that was devastating in its emotional intensity even though neither of us ever removed any clothes.

I was caught up in all that distraction, fantasy, pain, and emotional suffering compounded by the stereotypical conversations that included the phrase, "We have to stop seeing each other," which was always followed by (I can laugh about this today), "Let's get together tomorrow and talk about why we can't keep seeing each other."

It took two sponsors, a therapist, and an army of recovery friends to pry me loose from that relationship and to guard me while I "withdrew" from that craziness. It was like going through detox. I have no doubt that love addiction is a real addiction.

I understand why married men are a temptation. They offer proof of desirability—"he loves me more than her"—and instant gratification. A married man has no fear of commitment because he is still committed to his wife. It's simply endless rationalization and suffering.

Please know, if this is part of your story, you are not alone. Hopefully you know that the amends you make for loving a married man does not include telling his wife. No, the best amends is good therapy and coming to believe that you are worth so much more than that particular hell. And then, staying the heck away from married men—even as friends.

HAPPY, JOYOUS, AND . . . GAY?

"It's not that I was in denial about being attracted to women," Jennifer told me. "It's that I was in denial about how long I could deny that the attraction meant something."

We are having coffee and Jennifer is telling me about her marriage to a "very nice man" who she met in her first year of recovery. Her husband was also in a twelve-step program and they dated for a year before moving in together. "I loved the idea that I was becoming a 'normal person,'" she said. "I mean, I was sober, holding a job, and making friends, so it seemed that the next thing was to marry a nice man, right? So that's what I did."

Jennifer's new husband knew about her past, which had included some occasions of sex with women while under the influence. But he'd had a past, too, which included experiences that he was leaving behind for recovery. "I thought I could leave my attraction to women behind like someone else might stop lying or stop stealing petty cash at work."

Their marriage lasted eleven years. There were ups and downs as Jennifer and her husband continued their recovery programs, went to school, changed jobs, and moved to a new state. But, as she describes it, "The longer I stayed in recovery and worked my program, the more honest I wanted to be. I felt I could not hold my sobriety coin, which means honesty to me, while I was holding on to what felt like a huge secret."

After celebrating her tenth recovery anniversary Jennifer attended an out-of-town women's retreat. She heard a recovery speaker say from the podium, "You're as sick as your secrets," and her discomfort amplified. That speaker, who was a stranger to Jennifer, invited women in the audience who had secrets to tell them to her. "You'll never see me again so after the meeting please come tell me what you are holding on to." Jennifer went up to her and said, "I'm married and I'm a lesbian."

Speaking her truth to one stranger in recovery began the process that led to opening up to her therapist and then to a lesbian support group online. Thirteen months later Jennifer left the marriage and a year after that she met the woman who is now her partner.

"It was hard," she said. "But now I am fully myself and with a woman who loves me as me; we have a thriving marriage—we had a wedding a few years ago when Massachusetts legalized same-sex marriage." And yes, she continued, laughing, "I'm still not perfect; it's a marriage; I still have to stay close to recovery and communicate better and make amends when I don't. But this is the truth of me."

LITTLE KIDS, BIG KIDS, HIS KIDS, AND NEW KIDS

Some of us already had children when we came into recovery. Some didn't. Some had always wanted to have children and some didn't want the ones they had.

After many years in recovery and maybe several inventories, numerous amends, and some outside help, we begin to make peace with whatever our role as a parent is going to be. Some find the courage to adopt or become single parents on purpose; others become the kind of parent they always wanted to be. Some marry into new families and learn the value of the Twelve Steps for stepfamilies.

Those whose kids are experiencing their own addiction have an especially hard road. Being a parent in recovery and watching your child become dangerously engaged in alcohol or other drugs or any other manifestation of addiction can be painful. Watching your child—whether a teen, young adult, or adult child—struggle with addiction can be excruciating.

But there can be some good if you are in recovery and also dealing with a child with addiction. Having a recovery community and a group offers a big support to the parent of an addict. There is also the benefit of having some knowledge about the process of addiction and even of the way that addicts sometimes think. We might have less of a tendency to say, "Why do you keep doing that?" We know why. We have been there, too.

Watching your child—no matter his or her age—struggle with addiction brings particular challenges to a woman in recovery. It raises hard questions: "Did I cause this? Is my child struggling with addiction because of my genes or my example or both?" This painful time can also be a call for us to renew our own deep commitment to recovery.

I had a conversation with Sherry, who has been in recovery for more than twenty-five years. She had been so grateful to get into recovery when she was young and was able to be a recovering parent. She, like many, assumed this meant that her children would be spared her disease and her experience with addiction. But that wasn't the case.

Sherry's daughter was drinking alcohol and using other drugs. There had been interventions and even legal consequences, and there was also a brief period of abstinence, but Sherry's daughter was still in the thick of it. "I get so mad sometimes that I want to kill her," Sherry told me. "But then I see that she's doing a pretty good job of that herself."

Sherry talked about how being in her own twelve-step recovery had helped her to shift her thinking about her daughter's addiction. "I realized that over the years I had sponsored a number of women who came in and out of the program and I didn't want to kill them, so I had to remember that my daughter is in that same place as those other young women whom I have watched struggle. That gives me a little bit of perspective."

BUT THERE'S DANGER, TOO

I sat down to talk about women in recovery with Susan, who is a social worker and addiction counselor. When I asked her about vulnerabilities for women, Susan agreed immediately that there are both advantages and dangers for women in recovery when their own children are struggling with addiction. "It can be a dangerous time," she said.

"There is guilt for women in recovery when they realize that their child is suffering with addiction. They want to help them; they want to save them." Most women ask themselves, 'Did I cause this? Is it nature or nurture?' And the smart ones know that it's a little of both."

That guilt has to be talked about and processed. A recovering woman with a child who is struggling with addiction needs other recovering mothers to talk to. And she may need the help of an addiction specialist as well.

We know that the time when children marry or go off to college is a vulnerable time for women—there is grief and loss, and routines change. We have come to understand that kind of transition, but an additional time of vulnerability also occurs when adult children return home.

There is another time of vulnerability for women whose children are dealing with their own addiction. Susan explained the dangerous period when adult children come back home to live with their parents. In economic situations, with high unemployment, this can become more common.

We know that the time when children marry or go off to college is a vulnerable time for women—there is grief and loss, and routines change. We have come to understand that kind of transition, but an additional time of vulnerability also occurs when adult children return home.

What was once the "empty nest" becomes the "too-full nest." Young adults come back after college or brief employment and settle into their old bedrooms and maybe their old routines. They might have been drinking or using drugs in college or in their own apartment, and so they bring those habits back home with them.

A recovering woman who has not had to live with the presence of any addictive substances in her house for years now sees alcohol or other drugs in her day-to-day environment. That can be a relapse trigger. Adult children sometimes return home after a divorce or after losing a job and they may bring their turmoil, and possibly their addiction, with them. Even if adult children are not bringing drugs into the home they are often bringing their conflicts, struggles, drama, money problems, and/or their children with them.

When Stepfamilies Face Caregiving

This week I taught a caregiving workshop and had the opportunity to talk about another challenge of caregiving that some families face. It's one that folks will often wait to bring up privately after a workshop because there is still shame and discomfort. But many of us are in the large baby boomer demographic and that means that more of us are in or have been part of stepfamilies. We boomers have divorced and remarried more times than any previous generation. Those new marriages and new families have produced an additional "bump" of stepchildren.

What do you do when the ill family member is a stepparent or when caregiving for your partner involves the stepchildren?

There can be many complications. A woman may need extra help to care for her husband but his kids may resist helping a stepparent, or they might still have anger at their dad, or they could resent having to share caregiving duties with a new wife.

Every issue that makes being a stepfamily hard gets even harder in family caregiving: time, money, travel, decision-making, fear, and facing death, get an extra jab in a stepfamily. The standard advice about having a family meeting to make a caregiving team may not work if a former spouse refuses to work with a new partner or still tugs at the kid's loyalties.

SHARED RECOVERY

But there is also the possibility of an upside to this. When families do come together in recovery, the blessings can magnify. I spoke to Martha in Orleans, Massachusetts who, at age eighty, has been a stepmother for almost fifty years. "The relationship was never easy," she told me, "but then I had my little drinking problem too and that didn't help things," she continued laughing.

In recovery for twenty-eight years, Martha said that her stepdaughter was now in recovery as well. And, Martha shared, "I pass my recovery medallions on to her for her anniversaries." Martha's stepdaughter is sixty years old. While telling my sponsor about Martha and her stepdaughter I said, "Holy cow! I never thought about my stepchildren getting to be that old someday."

THE UNTHINKABLE:
WHEN A CHILD DIES

The email message was terse: "Had a call from Frank. He and Josephine leaving for LA. Anna has died." It felt unbelievable. Frank and Josephine were recovery friends. Their daughter Anna was eighteen years old. She was beautiful, smart, talented, and in her freshman year of college. Her parents were both in recovery for more than twenty years. She only knew them as recovering people. Yes, there had been the divorce when she was twelve, but this family managed that with high recovery standards as well. A mediated divorce settlement, shared custody, co-parenting, even Anna's birthday parties included her parents and stepparents and four sets of grandparents.

In truth, their home group counted this as a successful recovering family. Anna had been ill in her senior year of high school. She had been diagnosed with mononucleosis, which was explained as a consequence of stress. She had a part-time job and traveled to Haiti in the summer before college, and that September she wrote that she loved her college in Southern California.

One morning her roommate noticed that Anna was not rising early as was typical. When she tried to rouse her she realized that something was terribly wrong. Anna was dead. She had died in her sleep, a later autopsy showing that she'd had a massive cardiac arrest. The college police called Josephine in Baltimore to tell her that her daughter had died.

The unthinkable and the worst nightmare of any parent: A child has died. For a mother in recovery, like Josephine, this might be one of the times that any addictive substance or behavior could seem acceptable or understandable.

Josephine and Frank had to rally every recovery support they had—sponsors and friends and professionals. They were supported through the adrenaline-filled logistics and emotions of a wake and memorial service. Then the hard work began: remaking a recovering life and recommitting to recovery after this worst-thing-that-could-happen and the terrible void that it left behind.

The recovery habit of so many years, of using resources and friends, helped. Josephine attended the support group Compassionate Friends, which helps parents who have lost a child. She also found it helpful in that first year after Anna's death to attend her single home group meetings that took place every morning, rather than go to different meetings. "I could not bear to explain again and again that Anna had died and get those looks. It helped me to see the same recovery people every day and let them watch my feelings bounce all over the place."

Josephine explained that being divorced complicated her grief but that her recovery habits helped with that too. "Frank and I had to grieve together as parents, but he had a new wife, so I had to respect their boundaries as well. That was tricky. I talked to my sponsor and my therapist almost every day to sort out what was parenting and what was marriage. And when I did lose it, with him or his wife, I went right back to make some kind of amends, as messy as all that was."

Five years later Josephine is still grieving though it is less intense. Josephine is able to bring her experience to others who have experienced the death of a child, and when she tells her recovery story now, she talks about Anna and living through the year of her death. Newcomers always pay attention. Her story is clear evidence that we can go through overwhelmingly difficult experiences in recovery and not use.

MY FAVORITE RELATIONSHIP ADVICE

One of the top reasons for continuing attendance at meetings is that I get to hear the best advice and wisdom in those rooms. We get to borrow from others what it might take us years to distill on our own. A few weeks ago I heard a useful piece of relationship advice. This quickly grabbed my attention and gave me a way to see if I'm being reasonable when I start wanting my partner to change.

The advice was this: You can ask a partner for a behavior change but not a personality change. You can ask for behaviors you want from your partner but you can't ask them to be a different person inside—or to think like you do.

Here's an example: You can ask him to take a turn doing the laundry or you can ask him to clean the bathroom on Saturdays; those are behaviors. But you can't ask him to *care* about the bathroom being dirty or if you need socks; those are aspects of personality. You can ask him to buy and mail his sister's birthday gift (but please, please do not comment on what he chooses, don't sabotage yourself). But you can't ask him, "Why don't you remember your family's birthdays?" That is personality.

Similarly, you can say, "I'd like you to give me one compliment each day." That's a behavior. But it's not okay to say, "Why don't you appreciate me?" That's personality (and a good way to start a fight). Asking someone to change his or her personality is pretty much like saying, "Why don't you be me?" And would I ever want to be married to me? I don't think so.

Here's another helpful line heard in a meeting that helps me still, "If you want to kill a relationship outright, have an affair. But if you want to slowly bludgeon it to death, use criticism." And the longer I am married the more I need to remember that. The more comfortable we get, the more we feel free to correct, advise and, well . . . criticize.

Another piece of relationship advice I learned over these years of attending meetings is to "make your relationship emotionally safe." This, too, is something that I had to learn, forget, relearn, and keep practicing. Emotional safety is the primary necessity for a happy marriage. This, of course, explains many of the relationships that don't seem to make sense when we look at them from the outside. "Why are they together?" and "What does he/she see in him/her?" A man and a woman seem like they would never fit but what we may not see is the emotional safety they've created for each other.

In many relationships partners can't relax in every respect; they can't be themselves or realize their potential; they live with a constant of some degree of fear. A man or woman might put limits on his or her partner's growth or change. It might be unspoken and mutual, "Please stay the same so I don't have to feel uncomfortable." But without emotional safety, intimacy is impossible.

That's worth remembering if you find yourself complaining that your partner has a problem with intimacy. In recovery terms, we might ask ourselves, "What is my part in this problem?" Are you making it safe? No, it's not easy.

The big surprise for me was that emotional safety doesn't come from constant togetherness. Rather, partners feel safe when they relate to each other in ways that give pleasure such as speaking in a gentle tone of voice, respecting the partner's needs, not keeping score, and most importantly, laughing together. Shared jokes are more important than shared orgasms in creating intimacy and longevity.

TWIGS FOR CHAPTER SIX:
Love and Romance Later

- Together a long time? Take your partner on a date. You make all the romantic arrangements.

- Single and looking? Check out recovery activities for singles—cruises, classes, or sports. Google is your guide.

- Do you have a child struggling with addiction? Are you a stepparent? Try some Al-Anon or Nar-Anon— six meetings. It's all about detachment.

Chapter Seven

TAKE THIS JOB and LOVE IT

"LOVE AND WORK," SIGMUND FREUD said, "are the cornerstones of our humanness." Our life's challenge is in those words. With love, our task is to balance autonomy and intimacy. In other words, can I join with another person and remain myself? Similarly with work, we have to choose a perspective: Is work a joy or a punishment? It's a biblical dilemma. When Adam was banished from the Garden of Eden he was sentenced to labor all his days. That would suggest work as a bad thing. But in Proverbs there is the line with profound meaning, *Laborare est Orare*, "to work is to pray," signifying that our work is something holy.

In our contemporary recovery language, we remind each other to "practice the principles in all of our affairs," even at work. The skills we learned in recovery meetings—public speaking, meeting facilitation, and how to get along with different kinds of people—also help us on the job. In later recovery many of us go back to school or retool for new careers. We seek our "mission," we want to know God's will for us in work, and we wonder if we have a calling. We see some people turn hobbies into businesses and other people in recovery may leave big jobs in order to simplify their lives. Living a life of rigorous honesty makes us better employees. And practicing the Tenth-Step axiom of "When I am disturbed there is something I need to attend to in myself," teaches us to attend to our side of the street while on the job.

Years ago I read an article in the *Grapevine* (the magazine of Alcoholics Anonymous) in which the writer told of how he applied recovery principles to his job. His sponsor, tired of hearing the complaints about work, suggested that the man bring the same attitude he had for service at his home group into his role where he worked.

He began to see his tasks at work in the same light as making coffee, setting up chairs, or being treasurer. He began to show up at work each day reminding himself to "be of service." His attitude toward his work and toward his coworkers started to change. And he changed. I borrowed his idea and now I try to bring that same attitude to my work.

In recovery we talk about "practicing these principles in all of our affairs." And we try. We really do. After many years of recovery we learn that recovery matters most *outside* of meetings. We most often come up short with the people we love, and we also get to practice the principles of recovery at work.

Many of us change jobs, and sometimes careers, in these years. Going back to school is not uncommon. It's a consequence of learning more about ourselves. We choose new careers and new fields, based on who we now know we are and what we know we like, rather than what would please or impress someone else.

We discover whether we're good at math or we hate teaching or we always loved history or never knew we could write. Our sponsors and our home groups witness the transformation. First it's taking a noncredit photography class, and then building a darkroom, and later we enter a local photo contest and then one day we casually refer to ourselves as a photographer.

We choose new careers and new fields, based on who we now know we are and what we know we like, rather than what would please or impress someone else.

We have the benefit of a successful model for career development that comes from practicing "one-day-at-a-time" and "chunking it down" or breaking a big task into bite-sized pieces. That is the way we learned to do all that we want to do in our twelve-step programs.

SUCCESS AND FAILURE

Success and failure are both part of our recovery. One big surprise is that success can be as difficult as failure, and that failures can happen to women who have strong recovery. We survive both. And both success and failure offer us important growth experiences.

It seems to go like this: If, before recovery, you had a lot of failures in your life or work, then your task in recovery will be to deal with success. If you were one of those who always looked good on the outside, were always successful despite your addiction, then your "growth opportunity" in recovery may be to experience failure. I know that seems unfair, but I've seen it play out that way. Recovery and life have a way of balancing us out and of giving us the challenges we may have missed.

I remember working with a therapist early on in my recovery and I was constantly talking about my fear of getting fired, even though I had never been fired. In fact, I was getting promotions each year. I always felt as if everything was going to crash. It was the fear that I was going to be "found out," you know, that whole imposter/fraud-syndrome thing.

After many sessions of her listening to me continue to express my fear and her continuing to try to change my negative thinking, one day she finally said, "Maybe you will get fired." I was stunned; I felt terror. "Maybe," she continued, "you'll get fired and then you'll find out that it's not the end of the world." I wanted to kill her, and then myself. But I understood what she meant.

The flip side of failure is success. We can fear that too. You'd think that success wouldn't be a problem in recovery, but it can be an issue. This is especially true if we have not experienced success before. Like many recovering people, I had wasted my early college experiences. In recovery, I went back to school and day by day, one class at a time, I began to do well. My home group listened to me worry over each paper and they cheered each good grade.

Our recovery groups can re-parent us. When our sponsors and recovery friends nod approvingly at our first class, first test, and first good grade, it's like having parents who tape our vulnerable inner child's crayoned picture to the fridge. But there is also a painful reconciling with success in recovery. I was happy to be back in school and doing well, but seeing myself do well forced me to face the losses that went before— the opportunities I'd squandered, not because I wasn't smart, but because I had been living deep in my addiction.

We have to be careful with success, too. We get to experience our dreams and goals because of our recovery, but sometimes the achievement of those dreams and goals can take us right out of the rooms.

There are other kinds of success that can take a toll in recovery. Sometimes we get on a roll and realize that we can work hard and do well and the results add up. I've seen recovery friends go after more work, bigger jobs, new titles, all because they had the ability to do it now.

With a clear head, healthy energy, and the ability to focus, which they didn't have before, they began to chase work and career and financial dreams and saw them realized. Then they had to reconcile that with balance in a recovery life.

We have to be careful with success, too. We get to experience our dreams and goals because of our recovery, but sometimes the achievement of those dreams and goals can take us right out of the rooms.

In some situations it's hard to say whether an experience is a success or a failure. When I was fifteen years into recovery, and working at a nice job, I was invited to apply for a new job with a much fancier title. I liked the people I was working with at the time and it was a good organization, but the next rung on the ladder was right in front of me. I wanted the title of Executive Director.

I interviewed and was offered the job. My pride stepped up and I thought, *Yes, this is supposed to be mine.*

I arrived at the new job a few weeks later and I was thrilled. I had the title I'd dreamed of and an eager team of coworkers. However, in my third week on the job, the bookkeeper came to me and said there was no money. The sales that were in the pipeline hadn't materialized; the company had more debt than I'd guessed; and there were no immediate prospects for income. I felt crazy with fear and shame. Why hadn't I looked at the financials more carefully? Was I naive about the industry? Was I too impressed by the title to learn how to actually operate the company? People were still congratulating me on my new job when I made the decision to leave it. The other staff had the capability to produce income so I knew that I had to eliminate my position and lay myself off.

Yes, I felt bad. I felt extremely bad, like a total failure. I also feared it was a sign of my less-than-perfect recovery and that God was punishing me for indulging my ego that only weeks before had enjoyed the limelight.

It took five months to get a new job, and in the meantime I collected unemployment. But when I wasn't crying or cringing, I was able to appreciate the people who came forward to help me. People offered job leads and references and told me that this experience would certainly turn out to be something good. It did, but not for a long time. Years later, I was able to help another woman who found herself in an almost identical situation.

BEING A TEMP FOR GOD

The other thing that helped me with bringing my recovery into the workplace is what I call "being a temp for God."

This came to me when I was working at an organization that hired temporary employees from an employment agency to get through busy times. I noticed that most of the temps were pleasant, hardworking, and willing to do whatever needed to be done. They showed up each day and did what was on that day's list. There was no sense of right, wrong, should, shouldn't, not-my-job, or why me? I thought, *What if I came to work like that each day?*

So now, when I remember, I think of myself as a temporary worker and that the temp agency I work for is "God Hired You."

In my morning prayer I say, "Okay, God I'm temping for you today; whatever shows up is what you are asking me to do and like a good temp I'll do it pleasantly, willingly, and without debate. So where are you sending me today God?"

THE TEN COMMANDMENTS AT WORK

Recently I tried another strategy to integrate my recovery principles into my job. About a year ago I read a book that suggested we each write our own ten commandments. I was wrestling with situations and people at work so I tried this idea. My commandments are informed by my recovery lessons. The following are the ideals I strive for when I'm struggling at work.

Of course, I struggle with other people, but most of the time I'm actually struggling with myself.

My Ten Workplace Commandments

1. Praise and blame are all the same.

2. It doesn't matter.

3. Be of service.

4. It's not about me.

5. Do the tasks and detach.

6. I don't need to be important (or in the know).

7. Get along with everyone (be that employee).

8. Be an employee who doesn't have "issues."

9. Feel what I feel, but don't talk about it at work.

10. Do my work.

Geographic Cures

In early recovery we hear people talk about geographic cures and we laugh at the folly of our thinking. When we were in our active addiction, and maybe in early recovery too, it was tempting to fall for the idea that if we moved to a new place we'd become a new person. The joke says, "Each time I moved to a new place hoping to be a new me, a week later the old me would show up." In those first years it was a good check on our motives. Would the new job, city, or neighborhood make me a new me? Would I eventually show up?

But, later in recovery, we can still be using that idea in a less-than-positive way. We might turn this idea against ourselves by hanging onto houses, neighborhoods, cities, or jobs, wary that any impulse toward change is old thinking creeping in.

This is one of those areas where we can be open to a new perspective later in our recovery. Sometimes our growth and the rewards of our recovery are going to call for a geographic change. And a good one at that.

There may come a time when the benefits of working a good program pay off in wonderful ways. We get a promising job or we fall in love, and it means moving away from the town where we found recovery. It happened to me and it was both exhilarating and painful.

A couple of years ago I moved to a new city about sixty miles away in order to be closer to a new job. I was excited about the job and the growth that it both reflected and required. But I began to discount my own thinking, assuming that this was simply a new version of the old foolishness. After all, I knew that a geographic change doesn't make a new person. But I was in for a surprise. It turns out that after some years in recovery, if you check your motives, changing your work or home can actually help you become a new you.

No, not a complete transformation, and no, not a whole new person. But the fact is that when a person committed to recovery does change part of his or her life, it does result in a changed person. It works in later recovery because by then, if we have been consistently working a recovery program, we have the skills to integrate our experiences, to observe, think, feel, process, and choose. Yes, I was still me a week after my move, but the surprise was that I wasn't 100 percent the old me. Some part of me did change for the better. Maybe I was 80 percent of the former me, but I was also changed and still in the process of changing.

It's a bit like New Year's resolutions; we laugh because we know that we won't become thin or spiritual or athletic because of a resolution. But it's also true that, in fact, most of us will act a little differently if we've made a resolution and in that three-steps-forward-two-steps-backward way, we do change. So maybe what would be heresy at one year or five can lead to growth and positive change at ten or more, including the old "geographic cure."

CAN YOU SAY THAT AT WORK?

Here is a mini-test to see how well you are bringing your recovery with you to your workplace. On any given day at your job are you able to say:

- I was wrong.

- I don't know.

- I made a mistake.

- I'm sorry.

- It's my fault.

- You're right.

PEOPLE OVER TASK

In my fifth year of recovery I was beginning to get a little more responsibility at work and I had to find a middle ground between accepting my own competence and alternately feeling like I was useless and a fraud. It seemed that I teetered on that line daily. The result was a tremendous amount of fear and a similar amount of tension.

I knew I had to use my recovery resources in order not to feel that my promotion was a mistake, so I started talking to my sponsor about work, something I hadn't done before.

Up until then I had talked to her about how not to engage in my addiction, and we talked about how I behaved with men and in relationships and also about my family, which I had begun to "mine" for the root causes of my difficulties. But now there were better and healthier developments at work. My employment had been one of the first visible signs of my recovery, and I was stressed. I also genuinely wanted to be a good boss and supervisor.

My recovery so far had taught me that I should attend to "cleaning my side of the street" and the Tenth-Step axiom, "Whenever I am disturbed . . . ." Whenever I had a complaint, my sponsor liked to say, "So what's your part in this?" I knew that I was the one who had to change my behavior at work, but how?

My sponsor was a nurse manager and she supervised a number of people. We were sitting and talking one day, and I was telling her about the people I supervised and the problems they had (which meant I was telling her about the problems that I had) and she said, "Give me a pencil."

I did so, and she took a piece of paper. She said, "Here's what you do," and then she wrote the word, "people," then she drew a line under that and below the line she wrote, "task."

I looked at that and said, "People task?"

"No," she said, "'people *over* task.' Picture it like a formula or a fraction: people are over task; you put people over tasks."

"People over task," I repeated.

"Yep," she said. "Whenever you are dealing with people at work, especially when you are in a hurry or you feel like you know what's right and you want them to hurry up and 'do it now,' you need to say this over and over in your head like a mantra, 'People over task. People over task.'" She paused to allow her words to sink in.

"What that tells you," she said, "is that the people are more important than the work, more important than any particular task you are so focused on. Especially when you really want to say, 'Just do this,' and especially when you do not want to hear about someone's weekend or her kids' party or the husband's funny story—that is when you have to say 'people over task' to yourself and stand there and give that person your caring attention."

Wow! I knew what she meant but it was a big turnaround in my thinking. In my naiveté as a new manager I was sure that my job was to get more done and more done faster.

"No," my sponsor said. "You will eventually get more done and with better quality if you first attend to the people you are now leading. It's people over task."

I still say that to myself at work. Sometimes in a meeting I will draw that little diagram on my calendar or in the margins of the meeting agenda to keep my perspective in check.

People over task. It was some of the best sponsor advice I had ever received.

CONTINUING EDUCATION

One of the more compelling parts of long-term recovery is that we begin to discover who we were (before addiction) and who we are (after recovery). After we have immersed ourselves in recovery we often find that we want to learn more about life and recovery or we want to try what we once loved again.

It's common to see people in recovery go back to school. Some finish high school; some get a bachelor's degree, and some will go on to graduate or professional school. Some folks try new hobbies to keep busy and they discover unexpected joys.

Some discover that they like music or dance, and soon they are taking piano lessons or studying tango. I've watched friends become excellent photographers, serious ballroom dancers, and award-winning painters, sculptors, and jewelers.

But how do we learn new things? Even with long-term recovery, we have some character defects or characteristics that interfere. As we "practice these principles in all our affairs," we can bring our recovery lessons to our studies, classes, and hobbies. And we can apply recovery principles to our new interests.

A few years ago I noticed that many older people who had healthy and vibrant minds were regular bridge players. I decided to learn to play bridge. I talked to friends and they offered to show me the basics but I quickly became frustrated. The old messages in my head intruded, *I'm dumb*, and *I can't do this*. But years of recovery taught me that I could do what previously seemed too difficult if I could borrow a few recovery practices and apply them to my new challenge.

The old messages in my head intruded, I'm dumb, *and I can't do this. But years of recovery taught me that I could do what previously seemed too difficult if I could borrow a few recovery practices and apply them to my new challenge.*

So I got a "sponsor"—a bridge teacher—and I joined a "community"—a beginner's bridge class. I discovered that I could learn. It was slow and bumpy but we laughed a lot and made flashcards to practice and played for fun each week. And I learned to play bridge.

Here are the recovery principles I apply to learning new ideas:

- One day at a time. This means one class, one hand, or one hole at a time.

- Have a "beginner's mind." Be willing to be a student. I don't have to pretend to know more than I do, or more than the teacher.

- And always return to humility: It's okay to ask for help. I don't have to be the expert; I can be a humble beginner. That, too, is living happy, joyous, and free.

BILL'S ADVICE

I still need recovery reminders at my job. One of my favorites is this well-known bit of guidance from Bill Wilson. I copied it out of the book *As Bill Sees It* and it's taped to the bottom of my computer screen so that my eyes will fall on it at least once a day:

"True ambition is not what we thought it was. True ambition is the profound desire to live usefully and walk humbly under the grace of God."

TWIGS FOR CHAPTER SEVEN:
Take This Job and Love It

- Take this big challenge: One week of no gossip at work.

- Try one of the free online skill and strengths surveys. Look at the many options at the University of Pennsylvania Positive Psychology website. Compare your results with a recovering friend.

- Identify the person who most frustrates you at work. For three days, journal about him or her asking yourself, "What can I learn from _____?" Then pray for him or her.

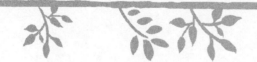

Chapter Eight

AGING, DYING, and DEATH

"HOW DO YOU GET TO be an old timer?" the newcomer asks. And the old timer answers, "You don't use and you don't die."

But if you are in recovery a long time, people around you will die. People in your home group and at your work place and yes, friends and family, too. All of the life circumstances that happen to people as they age will happen to people in recovery as well—physical changes, illness, disability, retirement, grief and loss, and caregiving.

We are privileged to see people in recovery go through serious illness, medical treatments, and even death. In my home group, a woman I'll call Sheryl showed us what it was like to go through a cancer diagnosis, surgery, and chemotherapy, another even worse diagnosis, and then hospice care. She did all this in recovery and actively using the principles of the Twelve Steps. She kept coming to meetings until three weeks before her death. She was our teacher.

If we stay in recovery for a long time, we will lose people we love. How we face their illnesses and deaths as recovering women is important. As we age in recovery, we have to learn what healthy grief looks and feels like. In this area, our spiritual practices and our growth in the emotional and spiritual realms meet their hardest test.

There Are Only Two Stories

It is said that there are only two stories, "A man goes on a journey," and "A stranger comes to town." Sometimes when I am talking to people who are new to caregiving, I might ask them, "Which one is your story?" There is no right answer, of course. Illnesses like cancer, cardiopulmonary disease, and Alzheimer's are journeys. They are shared and separate journeys depending on whether you are the patient or the caregiver. And at the same time, cancer, and dementia, and serious disabilities are also like strangers who have come to town.

In my thirty years of recovery I have lost many family members. I lived through the deaths of my parents and then of my two sisters and two brothers. I've had to face the confusing stages of grief and make sense of loss and pain in the context of recovery. I know now, having finally gone back to read her whole text, that the error I made about Elizabeth Kübler-Ross and grief was in taking her theories about grief in the abstract. The magazine synopses of her approach to grief often list the stages as denial, bargaining, anger, depression, and the end point, acceptance. But it is a misinterpretation to create the expectation of five discrete steps. And Kübler-Ross herself has been quoted as saying she is sorry that her original work gave the impression that there were, or that they happened in a particular order, or that all of them appeared in every case. However, they do serve as general guidelines.

This listing and numbering implies a kind of order, and that a person can move from point A to point B and get to the end and be all done. To those who have not been through this, it might seem like a kind of emotional Monopoly game where you go around the board in one direction, collect points, and then get to a distinct and certain end. This false notion of linearity is apparent when I hear people judge someone who is grieving, "Oh, she missed the anger stage," or "He has not yet reached acceptance."

I remember when I was in the first grade, learning about the United States from one of those wall-sized maps that were common in elementary classrooms, the ones that show each state as a different color, and I remember the first time we went on a family vacation to another state—how disappointed I was that all that distinguished the next state was a sign saying, "Welcome to Ohio." Where was the blue landscape my classroom map had shown? I was older, but similarly disappointed, when, after my oldest sister died, I discovered that the stages of grief that I'd heard about were not clearly delineated.

My grief did not move from clear stage to clear stage to a finish point called acceptance. Instead I found, as most mourners do, that I could be angry and happy and sad and in and out of denial and find acceptance and then be depressed all over again. It was anything but linear. I believe it is our fear, our terror of death that makes us want to organize grief, make it shape up, get in line, and have specific, manageable moments.

But the truth is that, in the time since that dying began, my life has expanded.

What was most striking to me, and is perhaps most surprising, is that there could be so much life in the midst of so much death. At a time when everything should have been dark and sad, I also had days of sincere joy and good energy and curiosity about life. When I look back at those years as my brothers and sisters were dying I can see that I was living—not merely surviving. Yes, there were times when my prayers were for survival—theirs, yes, but mostly and selfishly mine; I thought I would not, could not, survive the repeated blows of illness after illness and funeral after funeral.

But the truth is that, in the time since that dying began, my life has expanded. In these years during and through hospitals and funeral homes and cemeteries, I traveled, studied, made a new home, fell in love, and found good work. I also began to write, which was a long and secret dream. And I continued to grow in my recovery. It's as if I was opened to life.

THE GIFTS OF DEATH

We know that recovery has many paradoxes. That's also true when we are facing grief and loss.

"It was a gift." I've heard people say that when someone dies after a long illness. Sometimes we say it's a gift when spouses die together or a mother dies with her children, "Such a gift—she would have hated living." In these cases, we are suggesting a compensatory kind of gift, but there is another gift of death and grief that is rarely mentioned. It may be that the psychologists who write about grieving don't cover this because no one goes back to their grief counselor five years later to say, "I just can't get over this joy."

I am talking about joy as part of the grieving process. It seems a sacrilege to some, I know, and I have been through this enough to know that people have strong feelings about how mourners should feel, and if you don't conform to the prescribed sad, bad blues of grief, then you may be considered bad or mad. It does seem like a horror to admit that joy follows death, but it's true. It comes with a cracking open effect that grief has on us.

IN SICKNESS AND IN POOR HEALTH

The punch line to the old-timer's joke is, "You don't use and you don't die." But we are human beings and the truth is that while we may not use again, we will, in time, die. The only health statistic that is absolutely valid: 100 percent of people who are alive will die. Yes, even people with good recovery. So to paraphrase another recovery saying, the further you are from the last time you used, the closer you are to—yeah, dying.

We may want to deny this fact, but we of all people have learned enough about denial over these many years to understand that denial doesn't help us live better lives. Knowing and accepting the inevitability of death can help us live a better life. It can help us to know ourselves and make good choices now, in this moment.

So how do we live with and manage the health problems, the illnesses, injuries, and the chronic conditions that come with aging? There is nothing shiny and sparkly about this part of long-term recovery, but facing it can offer some powerful spiritual growth. Confronting these situations allows us to experience some definitive and concrete measures of just how sober we are.

One of the reasons I keep going to meetings is unquestionably selfish. Over these almost thirty years, I have heard so many stories and seen so many people deal with devastatingly hard situations—all while not using their addiction as a way to cope. That's a daily reminder that the ordinary and even difficult blows of daily life are no reason to eat or use alcohol or other drugs or engage in any other addictive behaviors. But it's also a reminder that tells me to stay in shape, spiritually and emotionally, because I want to go through the hard times in my life as a recovering and relatively sane woman.

The difficulties that we see folks go through are the illnesses of children, spouses, parents, siblings, and friends. We see our recovery colleagues in twelve-step rooms deal with cancer, heart disease, and dementia. We watch them live with injuries and illnesses that improve, and we also see them struggle with disabilities and illnesses that worsen over time. We watch our recovery friends confront and deal with death. We see people face the deaths of the people they love, and also, finally, their own deaths. That, I think, is like the graduate school of long-term recovery, or rather, recovery without bounds.

I've always been a worrier, so I have to balance this idea of preparation with the fact that we can never be fully prepared. As a kid in a challenging family, I developed the "what if . . ." habit. It was a strange kind of comfort, I suppose. As a powerless child, I could mentally rehearse the bad possibilities that might happen and it gave me an illusion of control.

I've always been a worrier, so I have to balance this idea of preparation with the fact that we can never be fully prepared.

But maybe now I can keep recovery at the center of my life so that I am prepared for those inevitable challenges. I can prepare my mind and spirit, so that when illness or death shows up, I can deal with it as a loving, recovering woman.

WE'RE THE JAM IN THE SANDWICH

About a year ago I was in Toronto browsing in a shoe store. I began eavesdropping on a mother and daughter who were shopping for shoes. It brought back memories. What I heard was this:

One said, "I don't care what you like; we're not buying those, try on the other pair."

And, "For the party you can get what you like, but we're not buying those."

The other one answered, "Fine then," and let out a big sigh.

One is rolling her eyes. The other one slouches in her seat.

I remember scenes like that from my own teen years. I remember, too, having that conversation with my stepdaughter when she was a teenager.

But this is something else. This was a fifty-something daughter frustrated with her eighty-something mother who was angry and humiliated that she couldn't buy the shoes that she liked. I could see the pain on the grown daughter's face as she explained, "The doctor said you can't wear slip-ons; you have to have shoes that tie because of your cane."

On the surface, taking one's mother shoe-shopping is not new, but to be the one holding the credit card, and the one who is saying yes or no to clothing and menu and housing choices puts us in places we never expected to find ourselves emotionally.

It happens that I was in the shoe store that day because my husband had come to this city so he could meet with his mother's banker. My mother-in-law was more and more confused by her finances, so this day her son was taking away her credit cards and her checkbook, as he had taken her car keys a few years before.

It feels like we can track the progress of our lives as women by our shoes. Little girls can't wait to give up babyish tie-on shoes for big-girl loafers, then out of loafers and into high-heels, then it's the cool new sneakers, and back and forth until a grown daughter is telling her mother that she can't buy slip-ons.

It's an uncomfortable process, taking over our parents' lives. First it's the car keys, then the checkbook—with my mother-in-law, even the teakettle had to go. It boiled dry one time too many.

There is comfort in numbers. Seven of us turn age fifty every minute; we join the ranks of folks who live longer and have more needs. AARP reports that an estimated 22.5 million households—that's one in four—provide care for someone over sixty, while according to the National Center for Health Statistics, average life expectancy has risen, from sixty-nine years in 1960 to seventy-nine years in 2006. We have met the elderly and they are us—and ours. The generation that didn't trust anyone over thirty is now over fifty, and many of us are caring for folks over seventy.

We who are in this "sandwich generation" are squeezed between the demands of children and parents. We are sitting at the kitchen table writing one check for tuition and another for extended care.

But it's not only about the money. This uncomfortable role of being "the big cheese" for our family raises new questions and unspoken worries about care and responsibility.

It used to be that there was a pause in midlife between getting your kids out of the house and moving your folks in; a pause that meant adult contemplation and time to face one's own mortality, a time to focus and regroup for part two: life after midlife.

We live this circle of breaking away from parents, becoming parents, taking on our own parents, and then allowing our kids to parent us. Just as we had to back away from the ones we raised as they came to adulthood, we now reverse the process and intrude into our parents' lives and choices.

Past generations watched their parents die and learned what they wanted and needed from that close look at mortality, and then—ideally—made better choices about how to live their own later years. Now we face two retirements at the same time, planning retirement from our work while retiring our role of being children of our parents. Because these tasks have become compressed, we lose that breathing space between life stages. For many of us, it's simply tiring.

For women who are caregivers, this is especially trying and it can be a health hazard as well as a challenge to our recovery. Here are some statistics on women caregivers from ongoing studies by MetLife.

- More than 75 percent of all caregivers are women.

- The average caregiver is female, forty-six years old, married, and works outside the home.

- She has an annual income of $35,000.

Here are the workplace and career consequences for woman caregivers:

- 33 percent decreased work hours.

- 29 percent passed up a promotion or training.

- 22 percent took a leave of absence.

- 20 percent went from full-time to part-time.

- 20 percent quit their jobs.

- 13 percent retired early.

Caregiving also has a critical impact on women's health: Women caregivers are less likely than other women to have their own health needs met.

Again from MetLife:

- 54 percent developed a chronic health condition, and,

- 52 percent exhibited symptoms of depression.

Coronary heart disease is a physical risk of caregiving. Women who spend nine or more hours per week caring for a family member will double their risk of coronary heart disease. And remember, despite all the pink ribbons, breast cancer is not the biggest killer of women—heart disease is. Other documented risks for women caregivers: poorer immune function, slower wound healing, and hypertension.

Many of us commiserate with friends in recovery and we may let those close to us hear the ambivalence, that is, our fear and guilt that we feel about our parents, but there's another group we need to include in this care and conversation, our own kids.

The next generation needs to be in on how we are with our parents, not only because we need a hand, but also to wise them up about their future with us. We'll be living considerably longer too, and our generation, with its sense of empowerment and self-sufficiency, won't be going off to nursing care any more easily than those in their seventies and eighties are doing today.

We need to let the next generation see our ambivalence, not try to spare them from it, because the truth is we can't.

We can offer them the understanding that the pain that comes with this territory is built-in and that their own future reluctance and resistance when caring for us will be normal. We can give our kids permission now to take our car keys and the checkbook and yes, even the teakettle, when that time comes.

As we go through this "sandwich generation" process we could say to them, "Look closely, some day this task will be yours; someday this dance will be between you and me."

I Can't Remember; Do I Know You?

Here's an odd piece of late recovery that people before us didn't have to face. We are facing an epidemic of dementia in our country. Whether it is from Alzheimer's or medication or the result of a geriatric depression—there are simply more people living with dementia. And because of changes in family structures and healthcare responses there are more people living with dementia at home and in the community. Some percentage of us—yes, even people with good recovery—will experience dementia. It means that we will forget events and we will forget people and we even might forget some experiences or qualities about ourselves—like the fact that we have the disease of addiction.

What would it mean to forget that you don't drink alcohol or take other drugs or that you don't eat boxes of chocolate or cookies or gallons of ice cream? Well, you might think, "Who cares at that point?" But I think we would care. And this might be precisely one of the selfish reasons to keep a constant presence in meetings and in a program of recovery.

Keeping close to recovery means that there will be people who will know me and my addiction and who will keep an eye out for me, as I will for them. If my brain and memory are failing, I hope my recovery friends will suggest that I don't keep that bottle of wine that was a holiday gift, or who will remind my family or caregivers, "If she asks for wine, the answer is 'no.'" (And maybe slip into that family member's hand the phone number of a home group member or two to call for help or support, should it be needed.)

If my brain and memory are failing, I hope my recovery friends will suggest that I don't keep that bottle of wine that was a holiday gift, or who will remind my family or caregivers, "If she asks for wine, the answer is 'no.'"

'TIS A BITTER THING TO LOVE WHAT DEATH CAN TOUCH

Perhaps the hardest blows we will face will not be our own deaths but the deaths of those we love. If we have been in recovery a long time, we have watched others do this. We may have admired them and wondered if we could do it too. Or we may have seen people relapse because they were not able to manage the feelings or the depression that accompanied grief or bereavement. This is one of those challenges that certainly lie ahead of us if we plan to stay in recovery a long time.

In a women's meeting in Chatham, Massachusetts, I met Pat, who has been in recovery for twenty-six years. Seven months earlier, her husband of twenty years was killed in a motorcycle accident. He, too, had been in recovery.

Pat shared about using the tools of recovery and the Twelve Steps to deal with her grief. "I remind myself" she said, "that I am powerless over his death and powerless over my grief. I also pray to be restored to sanity as I proceed through my mourning." Pat talked about needing to stay close to recovery for herself and to help her fifteen-year-old son. "I want him to know that he doesn't have to use alcohol or other drugs to get through his grief either."

Many women in this large meeting nodded along with Pat. With a median age of fifty, the women in this group had lost partners, parents, and even children. When the time came to close the meeting the chairperson asked if anyone had a "burning desire," a special need to speak, before the meeting ended. A woman across the room raised her hand and in a choked voice she said, "I just need to say that the woman who was found dead in the woods yesterday was my cousin. We don't even know what happened yet and I don't even know what I feel, but I needed to tell you."

This is what we have when we stay long in our recovery program. We can't deny death and we can't stop grief—we don't even want to stop grief or any of our feelings now, but we have safe places and safe people with whom to share these hard, sad, and tragic experiences that come to us as part of being human.

Retirement Isn't All Picnics

It's true. Those of us who are still working like to fantasize about what we'll do when we don't have to get up early on Monday mornings. But leaving the structure of a workplace can often be a hard thing for women in recovery.

Many women get into twelve-step recovery when they are employed. So retirement is a big change. Years ago, most of us had time to plan ahead for retirement—we planned, researched, maybe tried out a new city on vacation times or saved up to buy a vacation home. But with the changing economy, even retirement can come faster than we can prepare for it.

Many companies decide overnight to restructure. A recovering woman might be asked to retire or be offered a severance package and need to make a decision with just a few weeks' notice. You can lose daily structure, routines, and an important role in the blink of an eye. Relationships change in recovery. One half of a couple might retire and the other still goes to work, or a friend may still be working, and it will shift the dynamics of a friendship.

This also means the recovery habits will change. Meeting attendance will shift and even geography will change. All of that brings big new emotional and logistical challenges to long-term recovery.

Life Changes Fast

There are times in long-term recovery when we are going along and living our lives and we may wonder, "Is this all there is?" We might even feel, after years of recovery, that we are a little bit in control, that we can plan the future. And then something happens and we remember, shockingly, that life can change abruptly.

It's one of those parts of life we understand intellectually but don't grasp until it happens. For some of us this became clear on September 11, 2001. Others experienced it five years later in the London bombings. In many parts of the world there are incidents and moments when, as much as we believe in a linear life and invest in planning, we are shown again that life changes fast.

We know it happens. We watch the news. We know intellectually that change—via political upheaval or natural cataclysm—happens instantly and without warning. We almost expect it in other places or cultures. But it most often occurs closer to us personally, where the impact is always more intense.

Those are the defining moments, the moments that both build character and reveal it. Even as I write this, I am praying under my breath, "Please God, enough character already; no more growth experiences please." But they keep coming.

Last fall, a friend lost her home and everything in it—burned to the ground. All was gone—her checkbook, toothbrush, grocery list, computer, family Bible—not even a pencil left to make a tally of what she had lost. Her family was safe, and for that we say, "Thank God," but . . . .

In March, another friend was crossing the street. Earlier that morning she had been doing some volunteer work with a women's peace organization. She remembers stepping into the intersection, then regaining consciousness in an emergency room, badly broken. She'd been hit by a car and she had multiple injuries, the kind that take months of rehabilitation. What about the long to-do list in her purse, her responsibilities at work, and the library books she always returned on time?

I have always measured myself by my work, but last year that changed too when two organizations merged. Someone asked me, "What about your career?" and I answered— meaning to be glib but surprising myself with the truth—"I don't have a career, I have a life."

That insight didn't come easily. It had been growing over time and had been incubated by many funerals over the years and by many days spent in intensive care waiting rooms watching as most of my family died. That was a kind of wisdom school, the kind with steep tuition.

When my brother Larry was only weeks from death and we finally got around to talking about his reality, I took a deep breath one day and asked him, "Are you afraid to die?" There was a long silence. Then he quietly said, "Di, all I ever did was work." His words come back to me often.

We can't control everything, but we get to make choices. We can love others, allow ourselves to be loved, and say, "yes" more than we say "no." We can live our lives, because change may come quickly.

The signal may be a lone package left on the train, or a screech of tires, a drunk driver coming the wrong way, or a cough that won't quit. Or there may be no signal—only the realization (too often in hindsight) that life changes unexpectedly fast. The little Diane who tried to prepare for catastrophe has now grown up into a recovering woman who tries always to remember that control is an illusion, and the best preparation is to accept that change is inevitable.

TWIGS FOR CHAPTER EIGHT:
Aging, Dying, and Death

- Write a brief vision of yourself ten years from now. What are you like? Who is around you? What will your aging recovery look like?

- If you are a family caregiver or know you will be, make a file of local resources or take a Caregiver 101 class. Your local United Way can help you find that information.

- Does your recovery community have accessible meetings for people with disabilities or for people who are older? Can you help create that?

Chapter Nine

MIRROR, MIRROR
on the WALL

THERE'S A STORY WE TELL in my family about my niece, Sharon. When Sharon was a toddler, maybe three or four years old, her parents brought her to Pittsburgh for a visit with us. One of the attractions in our neighborhood was the Pittsburgh Aviary, a large and colorful glass pavilion filled with exotic birds.

One Saturday morning we took Sharon to see the birds. The adults spent most of their time visiting and talking while the kids wandered through the rooms of tropical plants. I was supposed to be watching Sharon but I got waylaid, and when I looked up she was gone.

I ran to look for her, hurrying through rooms of peacocks and cockatoos, and finally, I saw her in a room straight ahead. I stopped to watch her. Sharon was standing in front of a birdcage. It was the Aviary's talking parrot. He was no big deal; he only knew how to say one line. He kept repeating, "You're so pretty."

And there in front of the parrot was Sharon, standing with her little hands folded demurely in front of her, chin dropped coquettishly to one side, her eyes lowered, and she was saying over and over, "Oh, thank you. Oh, thank you."

I thought about Sharon's story recently when I went to a fancy beauty salon for a makeup lesson. Trish, the makeup artist, had been recommended by a friend. So I spent the morning swathed in pink, listening intently as Trish spent almost two hours going through all the tiny pots and tubes on her counter. Trish recommended a lip mask, special scrub beads, facial vitamins, and a four-part nighttime procedure. One hundred and sixty dollars later I had a made-over face, a pink tote bag of new makeup and some tricks to try at home.

After she had finished my makeover, Trish, and all of her coworkers—and even the lady who took my check—said, "You look so pretty."

I simply said, "Oh, thank you."

Over the years I've had makeovers in department stores and at-home skincare parties with friends. Once I even signed on for a high-end physician's line. I actually became a member. (The high-end physician wouldn't just sell me his special black soap unless I took an oath—and paid $175.)

I've even had my colors done. That cost $125. I was draped in silver and gold lamé while bright lights were shone in my eyes. After much contemplation, Suzanne, the "color consultant," declared, "Yes, you are definitely a 'Spring.'"

I emerged from her studio with a swatch book for my "Spring" diagnosis. That day I went to an outlet and bought $200 worth of cotton turtlenecks and spent $100 on scarves in my new colors. A one-day total of $375 for "Spring" training. So I am as fond as the next woman of experimenting with and trying to enhance my looks.

IS THIS A RECOVERING WOMAN'S ISSUE?

Is this an issue for women in recovery? I think it is. For starters we are women and we live in the North American culture, so we've been raised and trained by media and marketing to care about how we look. Maybe men have a version of this, but I think it's still true that men get ego boosts and life points more from work and accomplishment. Yes, career also matters to women but look at how those business success stories for women are written. Women are expected to be successful in their profession and look good at the same time. So, that's our culture and, in recovery, we are embedded in that culture.

Throughout my recovery, I have had an ongoing internal conversation that goes like this:

Voice One: I'm becoming a spiritual person now, so clothing and makeup and hair color do not matter.

Voice Two: But I'm a happier person now because of recovery and I am feeling good about myself; I want my outsides to match my insides.

Voice One: Diane, God doesn't care about hair color.

Voice Two: But God cares about beauty and happiness, so if being a blonde or having "warm" highlights makes me happy, what's the big deal?

Voice One: Yes, but . . .

And the dialog goes on and on and on . . . and round and round and round, too.

DRESSING THE PART

Even after thirty years, it continues. I've tried following each voice, sometimes to extremes, and then I let the appearance-pendulum swing the other way.

In early recovery I made a point of looking good. I made a note of what other women wore and tried to look like them. Where did I get the idea that there was a "recovery look"? From my own mind, of course. But get it I did.

In my first months of attending twelve-step meetings I went shopping for "meeting clothes." If attending meetings was to become a new part of my life, then I needed to have the right attire.

I had an idea that recovery would be kind of like Rotary or the Kiwanis: one dressed up, networked with others, did service, and there was probably an awards banquet at the end of the year. Being ambitious and self-serving, I thought I needed to look good to be a good member. (I also thought that I would figure out the hierarchy of this organization and take a leadership role, vice president perhaps, which would be good for my resume.) Again—what was I thinking? Well, you should know by now, I wasn't.

Then recovery did truly begin to "take" and I started to grow a little bit. That led me to my next phase of thinking, "I'm too spiritual for makeup and hair color." So for a year I was bare-faced and mousy. But I was oh, so spiritual! (I thought). Near the end of that year, I got a new sponsor who took good care of herself. In an early conversation, she asked if I ever thought about coloring my hair. When I told her that I had for years but that I gave up vanity for recovery she laughed and said, "Recovery does not mean wearing sackcloth and ashes— go get some highlights." And I was back.

Of course I rode that pendulum to another extreme, loading up my credit cards and having an annual tab at a fancy beauty salon that was more than what some people pay for their car—or their kid's tuition. So when I started to evaluate my money and finances, I let the "looking good" pendulum shift again.

A few years later, I was in the midst of a successful period at work. Promotions came and I was in a good job and enjoying worldly success as well as spiritual success in my recovery. My sponsor suggested that I go to a personal shopper at the local department store. The store advisor recommended that I needed a power suit, a silky red dress, and some good blazers for work and weekend.

She came to my apartment and went through my closet with me. (Think of it as kind of a sartorial personal inventory.) Then we shopped.

I did look good. The clothes were stylish and classy. But after buying all those shiny new clothes, I felt, well, a little too shiny. I found that those new clothes, especially the red dress, belonged more to an idea I had about myself than to my real self. So the pendulum swung again.

Back and forth it's gone over these recovering years. I have a nice wardrobe now and most of it looks like it belongs to the same person. My stages of rock star, tweedy intellectual, corporate-power leader, and cute girlfriend have gradually integrated into a wardrobe that reflects who I know I am, most of the time.

SUIT UP AND SHOW UP

All of my life I had medicated with substances—food, booze, drugs, and always with a corresponding adjustment to my appearance, so why wouldn't recovery need its own attire?

Many years into recovery I heard that some women had sponsors who told them to put on lipstick and change their clothes to go to meetings, as mine had told me to get highlights. They were to look their best, to work recovery from the outside in. I suspect that for the addicted woman whose addiction got her to the place where she never changed out of her bathrobe or sweat pants that's a good suggestion, but I was of the breed that was overly invested in my appearance. So rather than learning to "suit up and show up," I needed to experiment with "come as you are," and maybe even "come at your worst" to learn that I could still be liked and accepted.

So what does a sober, sane, happy woman look like? She looks like her best self. Sometimes that might mean high-heels and highlights. Some times it means a face shiny with tears and the glow that comes from crying it all out.

RECLAIMING MY FACE

A few years ago I was on a month-long writing retreat. I lived in a barn with a bedroom and an art studio and I didn't care about clothes or hair or even bathing. I didn't wear any makeup for a month and I liked how I looked. But at the end of thirty days I began to wonder if I could go back into my "normal" world without makeup?

As I packed to leave the retreat I began to ask, "Can I go another week without makeup? Can I go two weeks?" I wanted wearing makeup to be a choice and not something that I *had* to do. If I can be in the world without makeup, then makeup can be a choice. Can I use makeup but not be defined by it?

When I talked to my sponsor I said, "I think I'm reclaiming my face." If this is what I truly look like, I don't want to hide that. I don't want to be afraid of my own face.

It's about aging of course. Many of us admire the freedom of appearance of someone like Georgia O'Keefe, but most of us admire her ninety-year-old, desert-artist face. Yes, I may be willing to look like an elegantly wrinkled woman when I'm ninety, but what about at fifty-seven and sixty-seven and seventy-seven? The face we fret over most is the *getting-old* face rather than the *being-old* face.

Maybe this reclaiming is more a reclaiming of my mortality. Face-lifts might make us look younger, but they don't make us any younger. Botox may make us look less worried, but it doesn't make us feel less worried, it simply disguises an even larger worry.

I wrote this in my journal a few years ago:

If I am not my clothes,
and not my house, and not my job,
and not my face,
(and not my husband)
Who am I?

And the answer seems to be that I am a recovering woman, and while the outsides will probably always matter a little bit too much, each year I'm caring more and more about my insides too.

FASHION SHOPPING SECRETS

Here's a quiz: Have you ever come home from shopping and left your purchases in the car until you could sneak them into the house? Have you ever pretended that a new garment was something you've had for ages? Have you ever lied about a price or pretended that a new purchase was obtained on sale?

I speak from no moral mountaintop. I was once married to a man with severe color blindness. He thought I had a small wardrobe, mostly brown, because every time he said, "Is that new?" I'd say, "Oh no, I've had this forever."

They say that appearances can be deceiving, and they tell us don't judge a book by its cover, but that same "they" also tell us that we make decisions about others—and they about us—in the first three seconds. That would seem to support an investment in book covers and clothing and managing our appearance. We are told in recovery not to compare our insides to someone else's outsides, but we must also learn to align our insides and our own outsides.

There have been times in all of our lives when we have worn costumes, and even masks. The power suit and the professional demeanor of the businesswoman, the attire and equipment of the jogger or the athlete, even the slinky, sexy intimates of the courtesan or vamp. We dress for the parts we play, and sometimes—intentionally or not—we cross the line, from garments to get-ups.

Recovery lets me wear both garments and get-ups, and costumes and plain clothes. And it lets me both care and not care what I look like. Today I can wear old jeans, a ratty tee, and my husband's flannel shirt, and tomorrow I can wear a navy suit and pearls and chic shoes and still be me.

We dress for the parts we play, and sometimes—intentionally or not—we cross the line, from garments to get-ups.

"What do women want?" Freud asked. And the truest answer is: A high-class, good-looking black skirt; shoes that go from office to evening; and a trench coat that makes you look both smart and sexy. At least, that's what this woman wants. Do *you* know what you want?

Kidding aside—what do we want? Here's what I think we want. We want affiliation, love, friendships, self-esteem, work that uses the best of us, and genuine leisure, not just a swapping of to-do lists from weekday to weekend.

SHOES FOR WALKING
IN THESE WOODS

Can there be a book for women that doesn't talk about shoes? There are lots of reasons why women buy and love shoes. Shoes are an easy reward, a prize, and sometimes a drug. Even when you have bad hair or a bloated waistline you can try on shoes. You don't have to look at your face or hair or wrinkles or changing body when you try on shoes. There's also a practical benefit: New shoes can quickly update an outfit. The silhouette of your shoes can take you from shabby to chic and from dowdy to daring. Yep, there are countless reasons why women love shoes. But what do shoes have to do with recovery? Does footwear matter when we are ". . . trudging the road of happy destiny?"

Here's a lesson I learned about shoes from, of all people, my husband's therapist. While we know that nothing can fill a hole in us that exists in the past, and that no lover today can replace the love that our father didn't give us, and we are sure that no woman today can make right the hurt our mother caused, still, given that we know all that, we often chase those specific fixes throughout our adult lives.

My husband's therapist said to him one day, "Sometimes you can save a lot of time and money by just buying the thing you longed for so much."

"If as an adult," he continued, "you can afford the thing, and the deep longing is there, then go ahead and buy the 1971 Camaro or the basketball hoop for your yard or the black leather muscle jacket."

When I heard that, I knew what I needed to buy. I remembered the longing of my ninth-grade year; that summer I sat in algebra class next to a girl wearing navy blue soft leather flats with lime green piping on the edges and a tiny bow in front. I longed with all my heart for shoes like that. I later understood that those shoes—Pappagallo flats—were a symbol for all the social class wounds and the family dysfunction I lived with as a teenaged girl.

How many years did I shop, and how many other pairs of shoes did I buy to fill that teenage ache for navy-and-green shoes? Why not go buy them? I could do all the therapy and inventories and write dozens of letters to my parents to exorcise the pain of my younger self—and I did all those things—but then one day I bought expensive, navy leather flats and I thought, *Now, at age fifty, I rule the ninth grade in my heart.* Sometimes, if the shoe fits, you should just go buy it.

SEARCHING FOR THOMAS MERTON IN MY HANDBAG

I have a favorite handbag that I've carried for years. It is perfect. It holds my files, a journal, two kinds of pens, note cards, makeup, and money. I love this bag. It cost less than $100. Did I mention that I love it? However, when I go to the mall to Christmas shop, I stray. I fondle designer bags. I pet the suede, calfskin, and dyed canvas trimmed with leather. One of these bags costs as much as a car payment. But I want one. It's lust.

Back at home I look at the books piled on my coffee table, bedside table, and desk. There are books about personal growth and about making a better life and about how to have a spiritual connection and at the top of the pile sits

Thomas Merton—monk, philosopher, and writer. He had qualities I want: a life of contemplation, simplicity and, oh yes, renunciation. You know, from the word "renounce." As in "I renounce material goods." You see where I'm going here? How do these two opposites coexist?

Consumerism is based on the belief that problems have material solutions. We try to solve our problems by throwing valuable items at them. We do it with bigger cars, bigger houses, and bigger jobs. But some of us also do it by "consuming" more spirituality, trying more spiritual practices or teachers or even religion(s) as "products" to fix our lives.

Count me in! Yoga mat, meditation pillow, charms, chimes, statues, wall hangings, necklaces—one silver and one gold—to announce my belief in God and recovery. I buy more symbols to proclaim my belief in simplicity.

Yes, we all use consumption to create our identities. But it's equally flawed to create a self-image based on refusing to participate in the dominant culture or by disdaining those who do. The fundamental error is the same: Whether we derive our identity from consuming or from *not* consuming, we're still focused on self. Spiritual wanting is still wanting.

So how perfect is it that it's a handbag I am craving now? I can look in my trusty, favorite bag—literally a sack to carry my identity—to see who I am. It holds my driver's license, medical cards, and reward cards for the stores where I shop. My cell phone address book displays the details of what and who matters to me. But sometimes I still think a new bag with nicer outsides will change the inner me.

Even in recovery, we live at the intersection of spirituality and material consumption. I am searching for Thomas Merton in my handbag and hoping for peace in my undeniably open human heart.

TWIGS FOR CHAPTER NINE:
Mirror, Mirror on the Wall

- Do you always wear make-up? Try a weekend with no face paint. Journal and talk about that experience.

- Never wear makeup, or there's dust collecting in your makeup bag? Allow a full hour and step up to the best cosmetics counter in your town and ask for help.

- Try a new look inexpensively: In a thrift or consignment store pick out an "I could never wear that" dress or top then take it home and wear it. Try this with a buddy.

Chapter Ten

WE KEEP SAYING THANKS:
SERVICE and GRATITUDE

So Many Ways to Say Thanks

OVER HER MANY YEARS OF work with the poor and dying in India, Mother Teresa became a role model for caring service. Often, when she visited other countries to raise funds for her hospitals, she would be approached by women and men who were inspired by her example. Many people would ask her if they could come to India to work by her side. They wanted to be of service like she was. But Mother Teresa would encourage them to stay where they were and to find their own Calcutta.

She meant that while working with lepers in India is hard and humbling work, it is not the only way to be of service. There is not a particular place or a specific group that needs help more than others. She also made the point that to be of service, you need to open your eyes and simply begin. The world is full of people who need help and you might be most needed on the next street over in your own town.

Laurie Colwin was an American novelist who wrote clever novels about relationships. She was also a terrific food writer and had a regular column in *Gourmet Magazine*. In her book, *Home Cooking*, a collection of her essays about food, she wrote about her years of volunteering as the cook at a shelter for homeless, mentally ill women. She wrote about making large quantities of healthy, delicious food for the women at the shelter. When friends asked her if they should start cooking at the shelter, Colwin said of her service, "You have to find your people." Homeless, mentally ill women brought joy to Colwin, but another person might be better suited to help young athletes, or aspiring entrepreneurs, or people with cancer, or women in recovery. There is plenty of need in every community and clearly there are plenty of communities in need.

In early recovery, we are told that "service is gratitude in action." We were prodded to get a service commitment and so we signed up to make coffee, set up chairs, collect the money, or recruit speakers. Through these basic tasks, we met other recovering people and we became part of a group.

Doing service in recovery also teaches us relationship skills, as we have to deal with both criticism and praise. Someone likes the donuts we bring and someone else doesn't like the way we make the coffee.

Later we learn about other levels of twelve-step service. Perhaps we become the representative for our home group or we join the activities committee to plan a holiday marathon.

If public speaking is our skill we might speak at a regional conference.

In later recovery, the slogan "service is gratitude in action" now extends into all areas of our lives. Having learned how to be of service in our twelve-step community has benefits beyond the rooms. All those years of organizing marathons and conferences makes it easier to say yes when the PTA or a professional association asks for help.

Our human relations skills, honed by our interaction with so many different kinds of people in recovery, allow us to rise as leaders at work or in the community. Years of speaking at the recovery podium makes it less scary to step up to the podium at a town meeting. We learned how to say yes in our home group and now we say yes to the Chamber of Commerce or the town council. And, in the same way we once sponsored five newcomers, we can now coach a team. Now, as we become more aware of other people, we can also be more willing to help people in our town or community. When there is a need for someone to speak at church or to chair the library board meeting, we say yes.

Some of us still bake anniversary cakes and chair meetings at our home group, while others offer service in nonprofits and human services. Of course, it can be tricky, and we always have to check our motives. We want to be careful that our egos are not running the show—the recovery show or the community show.

But while the words and settings may be different when we teach adults to read or mentor teens, or coach a special needs adult to compete in the Special Olympics, it is still gratitude and it's still giving back.

PRACTICING GRATITUDE

When asked for a discussion topic in a twelve-step meeting, the odds are good that someone will suggest gratitude. By virtue of being in recovery, we have plenty to be grateful for. We know that having an attitude of gratitude makes everything we face so much easier. But how do we get that to be a regular part of who we are and how we think? The advice I have been told and that I tell others is to "practice gratitude."

But did you ever stop to think about what that means? Exactly how do we practice gratitude? I've been asking people how they actually practice gratitude, and I learned some interesting things.

First (and this seemed so obvious), some people I spoke with described making gratitude a habit. It can be a habit like exercising or not eating sugar or not worrying. Habits are repeated patterns of behavior or thought, and we can learn or unlearn habits. I had never thought of gratitude in that way. I thought gratitude was a feeling that came over me occasionally, but that it wasn't in my control.

Not the case.

So how do you get a gratitude habit? It's like the old joke about the man who goes to New York City and asks, "How do you get to Carnegie Hall?"

The answer: "Practice, practice, practice."

Psychologists tell us that twenty-one days is a kind of magic number for new-habit formation. So, to make gratitude into a habit, we can do some kind of gratitude practice for twenty-one days to make it "stick."

When I teach new writers I offer them this "twenty-one day rule" to help them become regular writers—that is, writers who write regularly. I invite them to do a mini-writing practice every day for twenty-one days, or ask them to write in their journals for twenty-one days. It's the same with exercise or walking—commit to a small quantity of a new behavior for that magic twenty-one days.

One of my favorite stories comes from a fitness trainer who asks his clients to simply dress in their sneakers and exercise clothes every morning for twenty-one days. "Once they are dressed," he says, "most of them will do some kind of exercise; we have created the habit of suiting-up to exercise."

I think that's brilliant.

So to give yourself a lasting attitude of gratitude, you have to create a ritual—a habit and actually *do a practice*—for at least twenty-one days. Here are some practices you could try.

- A daily gratitude list—you know this one. But do it in writing so that the hand and eye are involved. This makes the brain imbed the new habit faster. Decide on a number: Three items each day? Or five? Or ten? And stick to that number—in writing.

- Set the timer on your watch to the same time each day. An unusual number like 12:34 P.M. or 10:10 A.M. is good. When the alarm rings, you stop and quickly name three parts of your life for which you are grateful.

- Expand that idea to your phone. Teach yourself to have one grateful thought on the first ring of your

phone. Later, let that grow to the first ring of any
phone you hear.

- At home—when you are shaving or removing
  makeup—begin by naming out loud one specific
  thing you're grateful for that day.

- When you throw something in the trash, tie that
  physical action to saying, "I am grateful for . . ."
  quietly to yourself.

- What other simple habitual gestures can you link to
  naming a grateful thought? Taking out your keys?
  Starting the car? Taking your coffee mug from the
  cabinet?

The more of these repetitive and simple actions you can
attach to specifics that you are grateful for, the stronger your
habit of gratitude will become.

MARTY MANN

In the book *Mrs. Marty Mann,* Sally and David Brown write
about early AA member Marty Mann who was one of the
first women in twelve-step recovery and a close friend of Bill
Wilson. After a few years of sobriety and a deep commitment
to AA, Marty was—according to the Browns—ready to do
more. And this was becoming a common and recognized
phenomenon in the lives of alcoholics in AA after years of
recovery. It's as if they look around one day and say, "What
else is out there?"

Marty has been reported as noting that it's what we *do* with our recovery that counts. Our recovery is not an end in itself; it's a means to an even greater end.

THE PSYCHOLOGY OF SERVICE

Being of service in early recovery helps us become part of the group. And it gives us simple tasks and direct experiences that boost our self-esteem at a time when it's usually pretty low. But there is another benefit to helping, volunteering, and being of service in and out of the rooms. Being of service is not only a nice thing to do, it is actually good for us.

Martin Seligman, PhD—the father of positive psychology —has studied the benefits of altruism for many years and he includes service in his prescription for good mental health.

In his program at the University of Pennsylvania, Seligman has studied men and women in monitored experiments for many years to document the curative power of doing good. Seligman says, "If you are depressed the number one thing that you can do to feel better is to go out and help another person." He calls it the "number one thing." That is striking. It's also familiar. In twelve-step programs, we are taught from our first weeks to "be of service," and we are told that any time we are struggling or suffering, we should reach out to help someone else.

ENVY IS A GUIDE

A friend called to talk. She was miserable. "I feel envy," she said, "and it's gross; I'm envious of someone's house." I listened.

My friend has a gorgeous house of her own, but I understood. Over the years I have felt enough envy to know its acidic pain and the way the shame of it can silence me. Most of us can talk openly of our jealousy or even resentments, but envy? It's embarrassing. I have a nice life, but I have envy, too, and it has little to do with having enough.

I have envied people's clothes and jobs and books—and recently their dogs. So I listened to my house-craving friend and I told her about my envy. We began to dig around to see what is under this. What surfaced was the belief that the house, car, dog—or whatever—could fix us. Maybe it would magically change how I feel and who I am. But oh, I have to keep relearning: You can't fill a hole that exists in the past.

Philosopher David Hume wrote about envy in *A Treatise on Human Nature* in 1739, stating that ". . . it is not the great disproportion betwixt ourself and another which produces it (envy), but on the contrary, our proximity. A common soldier bears no envy for his general compared to what he will feel for his sergeant or corporal . . . ." The larger number of people we compare ourselves to, the more there will be for us to envy. It turns out that we compare ourselves most often to our friends. That's what makes envy so painful to talk about. So what is it good for?

I look at my closet. I own all types of lovely items, but nothing in that closet has the power to deliver me the way that something I *don't* own can. Envy is a con man who tugs at my sleeve and says, "Hey, listen, only for a second." He points out what I don't own: the shoes, the coat, the sweater, and then he whispers, "You'd be special if you had that. Come on, one more."

What most of us want is connection and community, but we go to the wrong places to find it. It's always out there—always "other." Paradoxically, we think that if we already have it, it's not enough. Hence envy double-teams with marketing and we shop like addicts.

There is some truth to the accusation that advertising creates demand, but that's not the whole story. You can lead a horse to water, but you can't make him wear Hermes or drink Evian. The envy in me reaches out as much as advertising reaches in; I am at best a partner and at worst an accomplice.

What is it we're longing for?

One of the highest-paid TV actors and the star of his own top-rated sitcom once told an interviewer he owed his incredible success to the fact that his father had never hugged him—"even once." He understood that he worked at his career in television in order to be loved. Becoming an actor may be a convoluted route to take to get to love, but it's a route that intersects ours. Like that actor, we want love, but because we hold that card so close to our chest, the real desire is hidden—even from us—until envy sidles up and says, "If you had a bigger house . . . ."

Sharon Zukin, a sociology professor and author of *Point of Purchase*, says in her lectures, "The appeal of a shopping spree is not that you'll buy a lot of stuff; the appeal is that, among the stuff you buy, you'll find what you truly desire."

Maybe the antidote to envy lies in wanting less. Rousseau said, "Wealth isn't an absolute; it's relative to desire; every time we seek something we can't afford, we can be counted as poor, regardless of how much money we actually have." Therefore, if we follow Rousseau's reasoning, there are two ways to feel content: try to get more money or curb your desires. And since we're not going Rousseau's "noble savage" route any time soon, how can we curb our desires?

We could get lost in something bigger than ourselves. The traditional route is God or faith, but we can also lose ourselves in a cause or an issue or helping our community. We could transform envy into service and give something away.

The Fire I Did Not Build

"We have all drunk from wells
we did not dig, and been
warmed by fires we did not build."

I have kept that quotation on a card over my desk for more than thirty years. Every person—no matter how comfortable their life may be—can look back through the branches of the family tree and find the place where someone in their family depended on the people who came before them and built a "fire" or dug a "well." This was true for my family. We needed a lot of help. And while I didn't "get it" for a long time, I finally realized that some person or some kind of service was there when we needed help. I went to schools that someone else started, had scholarships that someone else endowed, benefited from social services that others provided, and then I came into recovery to a program that thousands of other people built and cared for over the years so it would be here when I needed it.

So as part of my recovery, I have to be of service. We all do. There are many ways to do it. Some of us do it in our recovery groups and we often—in later recovery—learn to extend service outward as well. In addition to service in our recovery home groups or regions, we also give back by volunteering and also, maybe most profoundly, by keeping a compassionate heart.

GRATITUDE IN ACTION

Our gratitude is grounded in having a life that has more years in recovery than years in our addiction, and more years in good relationships than bad ones; more true friendships and job stability and genuine ambition. Maybe one of life's secrets we come to understand later in recovery is that we can be grateful for everything, even what might be considered our "mixed blessings."

At Thanksgiving, many families observe their own traditions, including one in which each member speaks up before the meal and tells the family gathered around the table one thing for which he or she is grateful.

At times like that, it is usual to name good health, career success, or our kid's accomplishments. But we often forget that some of our best gifts don't come in pretty wrapping.

Here are some examples: There was the day you were running late and thereby missed being in the big accident. Or the day you got lost in a new part of town but in your wandering, found a store that sold exactly what you had been hunting for months. Or you could up the ante a little: How about the time you got fired—but at out-placement you found the work you have been wanting to do? Or maybe the person you wanted to marry said "No," and broke your heart, but then months later you met the "one."

You get the idea, but we can push it further. How about the time a serious illness knocked you off your feet, but staying in bed gave you time to recast your life? Or maybe the struggle to accept a permanent disability revealed a talent you didn't know you had.

Maybe it was the arrest for driving while intoxicated (DWI) that was humiliating and expensive—but that's what got you to change your life. Or maybe it was an emotional breakdown that allowed you to put yourself back together in a new and stronger way.

You can take this even further. What about the death of a loved one that was devastating, but that led you one day, in the midst of grief, to feel something other than pain—and you realized you could feel joy like you never had before and you could feel it *because* the grief had cracked you open.

These mixed blessings are not easy to accept or admit, and sometimes it is faith that is the gift. If we are in recovery a long time, it is almost a guarantee that something stressful and hard to bear will happen. That is simply real life.

Of course the highest level of this kind of gratitude is saying "thank you" even before the good part comes. If you've had some experience you begin to know, even while life is painful or unpleasant, that there will be meaning in it. And so we can learn to say thank you—purely on faith—even when we're getting hit hard.

REAL HAPPINESS

In the past few years, a dozen new books and websites have been published that claim to help us get, keep, or understand happiness. Happiness is hot. In the fashionable world of publishing and social media, happiness is the new black.

I read all of these books and sites. I dig into them looking for tips and techniques, but this tsunami of happiness leaves me feeling like I've eaten too much candy.

It does seem to be an American phenomenon to want happiness in this deliberate way. And it's not new; our Bill of Rights includes the phrase "The pursuit of happiness" and our dollar bill carries the motto *annuit coeptis* or "providence has favored our undertakings," so we do have a kind of collective sense of entitlement. But at this time, when our country is in tough shape with energy, environment, and the economy all teetering—is it happiness we want, or is it something else?

Some of the new happiness research looks at "affective prediction," which reveals that most people are not highly skilled at predicting what would make them happy. That has to be especially true of people in recovery. I mean, look at our track record of making choices to make ourselves feel better.

The studies show that, despite what we wish and hope for, we don't know what will please us in the long run. Yet most of us insist on looking for that crucial something, whether it's a new car or job or relationship.

It turns out that we have emotional set points and that people pretty much feel the same degree of good or bad with only temporary ups and downs that come from events like winning the lottery or losing a loved one. Happy people tend to rebound to being happy, and unhappy people return to, well, looking for something else that might make them happy.

If we reflect on the guidance of a much older wisdom author, we can get some clarity on our cravings. Aristotle maintained that happiness comes from the use of reason. That might sound dry, but I think he was onto something. If we stop to think through our desire for a nicer car, newer house or, in my case, more shoes, we can see our patterns at play. A line from my daily meditation book often catches me in the midst of my latest pursuit, "You can never get enough of what you don't really want."

Maybe we could add some salad to our constant diet of happiness cake, and add a pinch of Aristotle. We can use our minds; we can work and live and help our community. That should be enough to make anyone happy.

TWIGS FOR CHAPTER TEN:
We Keep Saying Thanks:
Service and Gratitude

- Do you still have the gratitude list habit? Commit with a friend that you'll each make a gratitude list for fourteen nights.

- Where are you doing service? Pitch in to teach the newcomer coffee-maker or show a new meeting treasurer an easy way to keep the books.

- A new mom in your home group? Offer to hold the baby or take the toddler into the hallway so mom can hear the speakers.

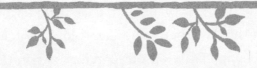

Chapter Eleven

≈

THE WAY WE DO
RECOVERY CHANGES

AS I WRITE THIS BOOK, I feel more and more gratitude for my recovery. I feel a lot of pride, too. Sometimes it feels like we're not supposed to be proud of our recovery, but maybe you too have spent thousands of hours going to meetings, and working the steps, and being a sponsor, and performing spiritual practices, and service, and therapy, and retreats, and inventories. I think we should be proud of that. While the healing may be a miracle, we can take credit for our commitment to recovery and for the time and energy and even the money that we have invested in our growth and change. But it's also true that humility will always find us (before we get overly proud of ourselves.)

WE ARE NOT SAINTS

Recently I had one of my "less-than-a-pink-cloud" moments. I think of these as the times when my home group members or even my best friend would be shocked if they saw me. I mean, here I am, a recovering woman, deeply committed to being a better person, and emotionally educated, and I am losing it. It's not pretty.

It went like this: It's about 8:00 A.M. and I'm getting ready to go to work. Once again I have made my to-do list too long. It's time to leave the house but I haven't put on any makeup yet, or made my lunch, and then I make the mistake of checking my email one more time. I see that there's a problem at the office. And then my husband points out the time—and he honestly *is* trying to be helpful—but in a second I am screaming, "This is too much" and then I'm sobbing. As I try to pull myself together, I think, *This is not what we tell the newcomer.*

But then I think, *Pray*; and then I think, *Change your thinking*; and then I think, *Move a muscle, change a thought*. So I go into the living room and—after I snap at my husband (like I said, not pretty)—I pick up a meditation book, which falls open to a page that contains this quote: "One of the symptoms of an approaching nervous breakdown is the belief that one's work is terribly important."

Bertrand Russell wrote that. I laughed out loud. I knew it was no accident to see that quote. And then I thought, *Well, maybe this messiness and this less-than-saintliness is what we should tell the newcomer about after all.*

STEP SEVEN IS A RETIREMENT PARTY

Here is something else that has changed over the years. The way I think about the parts of me that are not so pretty, like my "less-than-a-pink-cloud" days, has changed too. It's kind of like "progress not perfection," but it goes a little further in understanding and accepting the parts of me that make up the whole of me.

In the Seventh Step Prayer, we humbly ask God to remove the defects of character that "stand in the way of my usefulness to you and my fellows."

That was something I always wanted. But it took me a long time to understand that there is a difference between asking God to remove the defects that limit my usefulness to others and asking Him to remove the defects that I absolutely don't like or the ones I think affect how other people think of me.

And I don't get to use the Seventh Step in a self-serving way, "Now I'll get so good that everyone will like me."

I wanted the Seventh Step to be a self-improvement process or kind of like getting a makeover. What I have come to realize is that the deep change of this step is where humility kicks in. I don't get to choose the defects that will be removed; my higher power does. And I don't get to use the Seventh Step in a self-serving way, "Now I'll get so good that everyone will like me."

I had to learn to approach the Seventh Step and removal of character defects in a loving, as opposed to a self-bashing way. I needed help to do that.

One of my sponsors gave me this piece of insight: "We do not try to kill our character defects." She pointed out to me that my character defects were mostly the same characteristics that had saved my life when I was growing up. Being a "high screener"—having that super vigilance—was a life-saving skill in my alcoholic home. Being a super-organized kid (now I think of myself as "controlling") gave me a sense of safety and security in my childhood. And being able to anticipate other people's feelings and needs had made my chaotic home more manageable. Ditto with telling lies, stuffing feelings, being seductive or bossy, or complaining. They were all part of my survival. I had to accept that most of my defects were once my most important assets.

Until they weren't.

In recovery, I slowly got new skills of my own or I learned to imitate other recovering people's healthier behaviors, and gradually I didn't need that arsenal of "assets" from my childhood survival strategies anymore. My sponsor pointed out that it didn't make sense to hate these parts that used to work for me because they were, in fact, part of me. She strongly intimated that hating myself was not part of good recovery.

Instead, I could retire my character defects.

I love the idea of retirement. If we think of our character defects as former workers whose skills no longer fit our company's goals then retirement is honorable and appropriate. Much like in a business we can say, "Hey, we are on a new path now so maybe it's time to move on." But we honor the "retirees" for all they gave to our enterprise. Rather than shove our character defects out the door or pray that God destroys them, we could have a retirement party for our character defects.

Imagine that. We could have a little ceremony and list each defect and then thank it for its contributions and for its help in our early lives. There would be laughter and stories, like at a real retirement party. And then we could walk them to the door, take their keys, and shake their hand.

But we don't kill the retirees.

The thing I have to remember is that, like at any workplace, sometimes retirees come back to visit—and sometimes they visit at inopportune times—and that can be frustrating. But we don't kill them. We might say, "Hey, I remember you; I remember how we used to work together." And then, ever so gently, we might say, "But you don't work here anymore," and then we'd walk them to the door, and say, "Thanks again."

READING, WRITING, AND RECOVERY

Self-help reading sometimes takes a beating in the rooms of twelve-step recovery, but I'm ever-grateful for self-help books because that's how I got where I am today, which is where I like to be. Even before I got into recovery, I knew that something was wrong with me. The first place I turned for help was to the written word. I read advice columns and self-help books.

I know now that self-help by itself isn't much help if we are still addicted to substances or behaviors. But I believe that a smart woman learns from her own mistakes, and a wise woman learns from other people's. So I depend on and love self-help books and memoirs about relationships and addiction. Yes, please, I want all your stories. Tell me what you did and what happened.

In fact, I owe my recovery to a self-help book, *Women Who Love Too Much* by Robin Norwood. Norwood's book led me to the twelve-step programs I attend today to nourish my mind, body, and heart and to heal my spirit.

Women Who Love Too Much was so important to the opening of my eyes to addiction that I still use this shorthand for the title, "WWL2M." That book, ostensibly about relationships, also contained this challenge, "If you find yourself connecting to the ideas in this book, you may also have a problem with alcohol, drugs, food, or other substance addictions." I still have my first copy of WWL2M in a place of honor with all of my other recovery literature.

People say that no one gets into recovery because of a book, and that is only partially true. Many years ago a smart therapist helped me understand the value of reading this way: Some of us need to sneak up on ourselves in order to make major changes.

Recovery can take us into difficult places in our psyche and will require us to swim in troubling emotional waters. By reading about behaviors and emotions as we are working on them we can build a "cognitive life-raft," an intellectual base, on which to travel the challenging emotional waters that will lead to our growth.

So yes, books—large numbers of books and plenty of reading—are part of a joyous and long-term recovery.

I also find that keeping a journal is a crucial part of my recovery. I carry a small journal with me all the time and I keep a bigger one on the table where I do my morning prayers. Sometimes when I can't feel a connection with my higher power, I'll write out my prayers.

So while we don't talk about it so much in meetings, I believe that reading and writing are crucial to recovery.

A New Slogan

In earlier stages of recovery we learned, "easy does it, but do it" and we learned that "feelings are not facts," and we learned to "look back but don't stare" when we had to deal with issues of our past.

But last week I was talking to my friend Stephanie, who also has double-decade recovery, and she was telling me about something she does that undermines her happiness. I said to her, "Don't do that." Later in the conversation I was bemoaning a bad habit in my own thinking and was wondering how to change it and Stephanie said to me, "Don't do that."

So it hit me: "Don't do that" could be our new slogan. Whatever "that" is, we don't do it anymore. For example, don't shop with credit cards; don't eat cookies at 11:00 P.M.; don't say yes to volunteer commitments you'll later resent; don't agree to spend the day with someone you don't like.

After ten or more years of recovery, we know more about ourselves. The road is long, and there are surprises at every turn, but many of us know what makes us feel miserable, and for that we might practice this new slogan and simply, "Don't do that."

After ten or more years of recovery, we know more about ourselves. The road is long, and there are surprises at every turn, but many of us know what makes us feel miserable, and for that we might practice this new slogan and simply, "Don't do that."

ENVYING THE NEWCOMER

After many years of recovery, I feel shame when I do this. It happened again this week. A man in my home group celebrated his first six months of recovery and he was glowing. He shared how his life was transformed, how he had found a deep faith in a higher power, and how he had surrendered more deeply than he thought possible. He was quoting from the Big Book (AA's recovery book), and his "share" was more lecture than personal story, but I admit I felt envy.

I knew better. But I could feel myself become envious and annoyed. I knew that I should be happy for his pink cloud and changed life, but my own pettiness revealed my envy. After all these years and all this work, I'm still trying to surrender, have absolute faith, and be a perfectly perfect person. I know. I'm still, as we say in recovery, "shoulding on myself."

These are the moments when I wish for a twelve-step meeting held for people with ten or fifteen or twenty or more years. It's not that I want to leave other meetings behind, but so that I can say, "Does anyone else feel like this?" Is anyone else with long recovery secretly ashamed of their own petty reactions when someone with a year or so tells the group how perfect their life is and how they have incorporated all of the wisdom of the Twelve Steps?

I know better. I do. But still.

I'm sure I did this too when I was new. No, I know I did this. I was the girl carrying the recovery literature home to family holiday dinners and passing pamphlets around like hors d'oeuvres. I was the one who lectured every friend about the "principles of the program" and yes, I was the one blowing my anonymity hither and yon because I was so wise, so very wise.

So you'd think I'd have more compassion.

In my heart of hearts I do. I much prefer this new man be here in my meeting and feel like he's a guru than be out there drinking his life away. And I'm glad that he's lecturing us in this meeting rather than at home lecturing his family, which would only delay their ability to hear about this marvelous journey he has begun.

It's just that when I look at my own "progress-not-perfection" life, and I see the intractable character defects and the amount of fear that is still underlying so much of my behavior, I do have to fight my snarky inner commentator who wants to say to the perky, pastel-hued newcomer, "Oh, just you wait."

What I know now is that life happens to all of us, and that we need those pink clouds and happy days to give us the ground under the harder parts of our recovery. The pink cloud days help us make friends with others, including newcomers, so that we have a gang to hang out with, which means we'll have people to call when the harder parts of recovery inevitably happen.

My red-faced humility is this: When I hear those newcomers speak of their transformed lives and the perfect peace that recovery has given them, I still want what they have. So I keep coming back.

YOU GOTTA HAVE FRIENDS

One of the best and longest-lasting rewards of a life in recovery is having valued friends. It begins early. In the first months and years we discover that we can talk about ourselves with honesty and people say, "Keep coming back." We hear loving laughter and we are encouraged and supported, and even teased, toward more recovery.

According to Caroline Adams Miller, author of *Creating Your Best Life*, "We don't need a lot of close friends to experience well-being. In fact, having as few as four close friends with whom you share deep feelings and experiences is enough to inoculate you from stress and loneliness and to extend your life." In recovery most of us have that solid four, if not more.

Another argument for staying close to our recovery programs even after many years is that social science research has found that our feelings and behaviors are dramatically affected by our friends—even ones who don't live nearby. If we value their opinions and stay in touch, we are influenced by them, they are part of our internal reference group, and their impact is as powerful as those with whom we live and work. It's been found that not only are we more likely to gain weight if people in our closest circle gain weight, we are also more likely to quit smoking, be happy/lonely/sad, or behave altruistically if that's what our friends do.

So maybe a starting point of relapse-prevention is staying close to our friends in recovery.

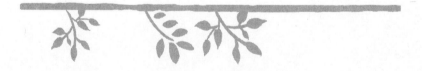

TWIGS FOR CHAPTER ELEVEN:
The Way We Do Recovery Changes

- Do you have a recovery "softball team"? Write out the list of your closest recovery friends. Are their numbers in your phone?

- How has technology changed your recovery habits? Do you text your sponsor? Have you joined an online group? Signed up for recovery messages on Twitter? Be teachable; ask a recovery friend to show you how.

- Do you have a favorite relationship/personal growth book, something that helped you with relationships or work or money? Buy an extra copy and give it to the young woman who is struggling.

Chapter Twelve

~

THE SCARY REALITY of RELAPSE and the REWARDS of REVITALIZING RECOVERY

IF WE TRULY BELIEVE THAT addiction is an illness, then we must also accept that, as with any illness, relapse is possible.

It's been said that recovery is like walking up a down escalator; it's impossible to stand still without moving backward. This is why, though we have much more peace and insight and good habits in our "out of the woods" lives, we are always in recovery and always vigilant.

Can we ever truly relax? Does having many years in recovery make us bulletproof? We know better. Yes, we hear more about "younger" folks relapsing, but it turns out that folks with longer recovery relapse at a pretty scary rate, too.

The warning signs of relapse may change with increased recovery. Typical relapse warning signs in early recovery are thoughts and experiences like denying our addiction, having physical cravings, and euphoric recall—that's when we remember only the positives of our addiction and what old timers called "romancing" (we can romance the food, the man, the praise at work, etc.).

It is no surprise that people with long-term recovery can be vulnerable to relapse if they do not monitor and manage the stress in their lives.

In later recovery, warning signs are more likely to be dissatisfaction with life, inability to find balance, complacency, and a gradual buildup of stress and emotional pain. People in recovery with busy lives, second families, divorce, or new careers often struggle with finding balance in all that stress. It is no surprise that people with long-term recovery can be vulnerable to relapse if they do not monitor and manage the stress in their lives.

WHAT THE STATISTICS SAY

A few weeks ago I read an article in *Renew Magazine* about relapse and it stopped me in my tracks. The author, Tracey Rauh, said that the accepted statistic for the number of people in recovery who will have at least one relapse in their first four years is 90 percent. That's stunning and scary.

But there was an even scarier statistic for those of us who have more than ten years of recovery: The more time you have in recovery, the less likely you are to return to a recovery program after a relapse.

That is daunting. If we relapse we don't go back . . . we suffer, struggle, and die, or even worse, we don't die, and we live miserable lives again.

The article went on to describe why people relapse from four chronic illnesses: substance abuse, diabetes, asthma, and hypertension. What they all have in common is that they are treatable, but if you don't take the medicine and you don't follow professional guidance, you will relapse.

The point the article made that struck me the most is that the more recovery you have, the less likely it is that you will survive a relapse. Read that again: *The more recovery you have, the less likely it is that you will survive a relapse.*

You might remember the saying we used to hear in meetings that goes like this, "While you are sitting here your addiction is out in the parking lot doing pushups." It turns out that this bit of twelve-step folk wisdom is true and statistically valid.

We hear often in meetings that the reason people relapse is that they stopped going to meetings. But I wonder if that is a cause or an effect.

As I researched relapse and longtime recovery it became clear that there are many people who keep going to meetings and still relapse, as well as many people who stop going to meetings and don't relapse. However, it makes sense that if you go to meetings you will also be doing some other important recovery activities that are relapse-preventive: staying close to recovery people, keeping recovery concepts/principles alive in your life, talking about what is going on in your life with people who are safe and supportive, and receiving encouragement to be honest with yourself and others.

My gut feeling is that the real issue around relapse has to do with honesty. The first triggers toward relapse, in my opinion, are keeping secrets and dishonesty. When we start to think, "I can't tell anyone this . . . ," whatever the "this" is, then we have a secret and we will want to isolate ourselves. We may be sitting in a room full of recovering people and we may be saying all the right recovery words and slogans, but if we have begun to feel shame, secretiveness, and dishonesty, then we are on step one of relapse.

Yes, we do live real lives and there may be situations where we have to keep confidences. We may have a home or work situation that we can't share with everyone. In those cases we talk to our sponsor or our partner or our recovery friends to get perspective. I have a friend who cannot talk openly about her husband's recently diagnosed disability because news of his illness could impact their business, but she talks to her sponsor and her therapist and two close recovery friends so that she is not alone with a secret.

In recovery meetings we hear that "You are only as sick as your secrets." The French say, "Nothing is so burdensome as a secret." But I know that the most damaging and most frightening secrets are the ones I keep from myself.

THE SILVER TSUNAMI

We know about the boomer bump. The huge demographic shift that is overtaking our economy and healthcare system is changing our family and social dynamics in many ways. Our rapidly aging community means more caregivers of all ages and increased longevity, but also more disability.

It also means more drug addiction and more misuse of alcohol and other drugs. The tsunami for older adults who are using and misusing substances is tricky because we have social and cultural blocks that prevent us from recognizing and addressing the issue. Can't Grandma enjoy her glass of wine? Why should Grandpa be in pain if his doctor is okay with giving him prescriptions? If the doctor says it's okay, what's the big deal?

But it is a big deal because we are seeing a huge increase in the number of people in their sixties who are first-time users of marijuana and cocaine. I know, seems crazy right? But Gramps is not down on the corner scoring the drugs from some kid, he's buying it at the senior center and in the assisted-living center lobby, and it comes right to his door in the senior high-rise.

The numbers compound when you consider that 10,000 people turn age sixty-five every day in the United States.

We know that alcohol and other drug use increases with stress, and that stress can be excessive over the typical two-to-eighteen months of a family member's serious illness. Better healthcare means that caregiving will go on and on and on and, well, who would deny someone in that situation some wine, or some Valium, or some Ambien or—if he or she is exhausted—a little cocaine?

Most folks over sixty have an average of eleven medications prescribed for them by an average of three doctors. The most prescribed medications for seniors are benzodiazepines, such as Valium, Xanax, etc. They are central nervous system depressants—and highly addictive. And they mimic the symptoms of dementia, so family, and even physicians, can be fooled.

Opioids are prescribed for pain. But chronic use can actually lower one's pain threshold. Chronic opioid use with prescribed medications can lead patients to feel more pain, a condition known as opioid-induced hyperalgesia, so then it seems natural to ask for and take more and stronger pain meds.

Caregivers of people with chronic illness are often living with significant unspoken resentments. Caring for a disabled or ill partner is not what they imagined retirement to be. Where is the fun? Where is the adventure they worked so hard to afford?

So naturally they might think, "Why can't I have a little wine or one of those new fancy drinks?" Boomers who may have used marijuana in their twenties and gave it up when it was time to be responsible for career and family, may romance the idea of being able to use pot again after their retirement. But the pot they can buy today is not like the drug they smoked in college—it is now much stronger.

Today there are specialized treatment services and inpatient programs for addicts over age sixty. And we can expect to see many more folks from the "Silver Tsunami" in our twelve-step groups as well.

A RECIPE FOR RELAPSE

Terry Gorski has written many articles about relapse. He describes it as a process and he says that relapse begins long before someone picks up a substance or goes back to a behavior to which they were addicted. Relapse begins, according to Gorski, with subtle forms of dissatisfaction.

So it's worth paying attention to the early warning signs. Here are Gorski's eight stages of relapse. It might be the basis for a weekly talk with your sponsor or recovering women friends.

THE EIGHT STAGES OF RELAPSE

1. Beginnings of secret dissatisfaction
2. Boredom or frustration at work or at home
3. Relationships change
4. Return of denial
5. Emotional drift (away from recovery friends, sponsor, supports)
6. Anger and resentment
7. Depression and dishonesty
8. Relapse

A key question to ask yourself is this: Are you abstinent or are you genuinely in recovery? People can be abstinent for long periods of time but they are never at ease or comfortable. They haven't actually changed their attitudes, beliefs, and habits. All that is needed is a simple trigger and they can find themselves back into using an addictive substance or behavior.

A Checklist for the Recovering Woman

Before we get too close to that final step and risk a relapse, we might want to keep tabs on our ongoing recovery. Here are some questions we can ask ourselves—and each other—on a regular basis.

Ask Yourself These Questions

- Do you participate in a recovery group?

- Do your close friends know that you are in recovery and that you do not drink alcohol or take other drugs, abuse food, etc?

- Do you read recovery literature—the old and the new?

- Do you have a sponsor? Yes, after all these years we still need someone with experience who will regularly remind us of recovery principles and practices.

- Do you talk to your healthcare practitioners about your addiction and your addiction history, especially when you are preparing for or recovering from surgery or cancer treatment or other serious illness?

- Do you talk to your doctor and pharmacist and sponsor about all medications that are prescribed or suggested, especially those for pain, anxiety, etc.?

- Do you keep anything secret from the important people in your life? No matter how long we are in recovery, it is still true that we are "as sick as our secrets."

- Do you pay attention to new or "transferred" addiction behaviors? Years after stopping alcohol or other drugs, you might develop an eating disorder, compulsive gambling problem, or prescription drug problem, etc. This is another reason why we keep close to a home group and to other people with long-term recovery.

- Do you continue to work the steps—with a step group, sponsor, spiritual director, or on an annual retreat?

No matter how many years we are in a recovery program, we can never forget that addiction is a chronic, and if left untreated, fatal disease. We can manage it, we can grow through it, and we do make new and better lives. But we have to be vigilant and never take our gift of recovery for granted.

A Recipe for Recovery

So what is recovery? What do you need to have, see, feel, and do to say you are indeed recovering? I've been chewing on that question while writing this book.

One of the best short versions of what constitutes recovery comes from Terry Gorski. If you've done some work as a recovering adult child (ACOA), you'll also know his name from the funny talk on recovery and dating he recorded in the 1980s. In my early years, we passed his tapes around and quoted his lines to each other—it was recovery stand-up, brilliant and funny.

I've gone back to Gorski's 1986 book, *Staying Sober* for his recipe for recovery, and here is what he says, "Sobriety is abstinence from addictive drugs *plus* abstinence from compulsive behaviors *plus* improvements in your bio/psycho/social health."

... *"So where am I in these woods and how is my recovery today?*

That one sentence is an excellent prescription for ongoing recovery. We could simply read his sentence each day and take a moment to ask ourselves, "So where am I in these woods and how is my recovery today?"

YOUR WAKE UP CALL

In early recovery I heard people say, "A little AA will ruin your drinking." Today we might say, "A little recovery will ruin any pleasure you might find in your addiction." The idea is that once you set out on this path to growth and recovery, you are forever changed, even if it takes longer than you expected or hoped to achieve abstinence. Your first step into the "woods" changes you.

Also in those early days of recovery, I heard the harsh sounding admonition, "Change or die." I remember being taken aback and thinking, "Well, isn't that a bit extreme?" I mean, I wanted the pain to stop and I wanted my life to be better but was I going to die? Now, so many years later, watching people around me choose to change or not—and choose to change *enough* or not—I know, and you do too, that people die from addiction. We have to change or die. That is, of course, what got us here. We were going to die, but instead we changed. Today, many years later, that's still the truth: We change or die. We keep growing. And always, we keep coming back.

TWIGS FOR CHAPTER TWELVE:
The Scary Reality of Relapse and the Rewards of Revitalizing Recovery

• Talk with your sponsor or someone who has recovery that you admire. Listen like a newcomer.

• Take the relapse inventory with recovering friends. Share your plans to address any concerns.

• During a period of quiet time every day, ask deeply what is next for your ongoing growth and recovery.